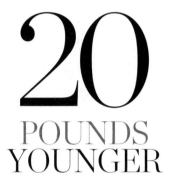

20
POUNDS
YOUNGER

The Life-Transforming Plan
for a Fitter, Sexier You!

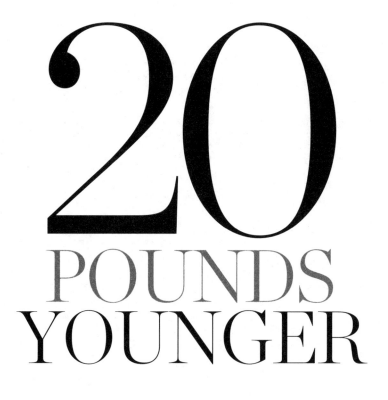

20
POUNDS
YOUNGER

Michele Promaulayko
Editor-in-Chief of YAHOO! HEALTH

WITH LAURA TEDESCO

RODALE.

© 2015 by Rodale Inc.

Rodale books may be purchased for business or promotional use or for special sales. For information, please write to:
Special Markets Department, Rodale, Inc., 733 Third Avenue, New York, NY 10017

Printed in the United States of America

Rodale Inc. makes every effort to use acid-free ∞, recycled paper ♲.

Exercise Photographs by Thomas MacDonald/Rodale Images

Book design by Kara Plikaitis

Library of Congress Cataloging-in-Publication Data is on file with the publisher.

978-1-62336-403-8

Distributed to the trade by Macmillan

2   4   6   8   10   9   7   5   3   1   hardcover

We inspire and enable people to improve their lives and the world around them.
rodalebooks.com

For every woman who wants to grow younger
and stronger in mind, body, and spirit.

CONTENTS

It Works for Me, It'll Work for **You**

WELCOME TO *20 POUNDS YOUNGER!* Just by seeking out this book, you've taken the super important step of prioritizing your health and happiness. And every action you take from this point on will reward that brave choice—I can't wait for you to see (and feel!) all of the positive changes that are to come.

Best of all, you aren't going to be on this journey alone, because although we're all unique individuals, as women we all belong to a big sisterhood whose members are facing many of the same challenges: to stay fit, healthy, energetic, strong, and, yes, sexy—which to me is way more about vibrancy and confidence than it is about a certain chest-to-waist-to-hip ratio.

This book is a powerful tool to help you look and feel 20 pounds younger, but I promise I'm not going to overload your day with unrealistic tasks. I'll respect your time because chances are, you're already pressed to do enough! You'll learn lots of effective strategies to lose weight, increase your fitness, reduce stress, eat healthier, and look radiant and beautiful.

I've spent a lot of time factoring efficiency into this plan because I know you are crazy busy, like me. But I also know it takes commitment to accomplish worthwhile goals. So the program we've set out for you is challenging but adaptable. I'll tell you what to do, with step-by-step instructions, but won't dictate or preach. It'll be up to you to figure out how to fit these tips and techniques into your day, because everybody's life is different.

Here's an overview of what 20 Pounds Younger is all about.

5 GOALS OF YOUR 20 POUNDS YOUNGER PROGRAM

1. **Eating mindfully,** because that's the big secret to lasting weight loss. And this book has tons of cool tricks to help you get into a mindful mode.

2. **Following a more healthful, antiaging diet** that will eliminate the taxing, outdated need to count calories. And don't worry, it's a delicious way to eat—promise!

3. **Reducing stress** and successfully combating the inherently female response of addressing anxiety with food—a cliché that needs to meet its demise.

4. **Exercising specifically to preserve your biggest 24-7 calorie burner:** your skeletal muscle (more on that later).

5. **Preserving and enhancing your attractiveness.**

Each piece of the program will give you practical tools and techniques that you can start using right away. You'll get Instant Age Erasers, and our top health experts will give you frank answers to frequently asked questions. It'll be challenging, but also fun.

Sound doable? It should be, if I've done my job of channeling your needs, which are probably pretty similar to my own and a lot of other women's. For example: There are few things I love more than eating a delicious meal—one that doesn't make me feel bad at the end of it. You, too? Most days I'm stressed out from burning the candle at both ends. You can relate, I'm sure. I long for the luxury of an hour of free time to exercise or to squeeze in a mani-pedi. Do you feel me?

Here's another universal truth: We can't instinctively always know what the right food and fitness choices are—we need someone in the know to show us the way . . . and to keep showing us the way, because health advice is always evolving. For example: In my twenties, long before I became the editor-in-chief of Yahoo Health and before that, the editor-in-chief of *Women's Health,* I followed the early-'90s approach to eating: If foods were fat-free, they *had* to be healthy, no matter how processed they were. I ate bagels the size of softballs because those carb bombs were fat-free, baby! Pasta, too. God, did I eat pasta. I'd guiltlessly make a meal out of fat-free foods thinking I was doing the right thing. (Nobody told me that the fat was replaced with sugar and other garbage.) I even refused to eat healthy fats— like coconut oil and almond butter, for example—because to me, all fat was equal (in other words, evil).

I just didn't know better. Growing up in a single-parent household meant that my mom was often too busy working to roast vegetables with rosemary. We were a meat-and-potatoes household; we ate precious few fresh greens (at least ones that weren't boiled to death). There was always ice cream in the freezer, soda in the fridge, and crackers and cookies in the pantry. My early years probably looked a lot like yours, and maybe your current diet still harbors some remnants from those days of eating out of boxes, cartons and cans.

Even in my late twenties and early thirties, when I was on my own— and expanded my palate beyond fat-free packaged foods—I still didn't know what healthy eating *really* meant. In fact, it wasn't until I started working as an editor at women's magazines that my perspective on food began to truly transform. I learned that "healthy" doesn't mean "fat free" or "low calorie." My jaw dropped when I started to recognize the hidden sugars in my foods and understand just how the sweet stuff affects your metabolism and weight, your arteries and brain, and even your skin and hair. Today, I can't look at a can of soda without imagining the 12-teaspoon pile of white sugar lurking inside.

I feel so grateful for the food education I received as editor-in-chief of *Women's Health* and getting to know the top minds in nutrition science. What I've learned has not only prepared me for my new role as editor-in-chief of Yahoo Health but has nudged me to improve my life in so many ways. Thanks to these healthy-eating pros, I've become more of a foodie than ever before. I'm what food journalist Mark Bittman calls a "less meat-atarian": I eat more greens, fish, and colorful vegetables than I used to, though I still eat meat, and I love fresh herbs and supernutritious raw food, too. I am and always have been a hungry girl, and I'm not shy about it. I'm not willing to give up avocados—my desert island food choice—just because they're high in calories (thanks to a generous dose of good-for-you fats!). Nor will I totally cut out fruit just because it contains sugar. And yes, I even indulge in ice cream from time to time.

As I've mentioned, I didn't figure all of this out on my own. During my incredible six years at *Women's Health* and my recent leap to Yahoo Health, I've had the privilege of learning from the world-renowned wellness experts—a group of people I lovingly refer to as my Life Stylists. This team of gurus has taught me how to meditate (something I *never* thought I, a total type-A person, would enjoy), to be mindful about what I put into my mouth, to lift weights for a leaner, more sculpted body (supplemented with a side of yoga)—and to feel incredible while doing all of it. I'll introduce you to these Life Stylists on page xx, and you'll benefit from their wisdom—just as I did—throughout the book! The result: I'm 44, and I'm in the best shape of my life. And I'm eager—and excited—to share the life-changing secrets that have elevated every part of me, inside and out. (For a sneak peek, check out my "10 Eye-Openers" on page xiii.)

So who is this book for and what does it promise? Well, it's for any woman who is fed up with typical, unsustainable diets. It's for any woman who has looked at herself in the mirror while wearing a bikini, poked at her soft spots, and muttered "Ugh!" in disgust. It's for the girl who's much too young to feel *this* old—tired, stressed, bummed out. It's for the chick who has woken up with puffy eyes and a bloated belly because she ate sushi (with too much soy sauce) the night before. Or had one too many cocktails. It's for the woman who lost weight and then gained it back with extra cheese and who compares her thighs to those of skinnier women and wonders, "What's *their* secret?" Many of these descriptions, thoughts and sentiments ring true for me, personally.

Let's stop with the guilt, for good. This book's mission—its unwavering promise—is to banish the negativity and self-blaming and replace it with acceptance, love, empowerment, and tried-and-tested tools that really, truly work. As the editor-in-chief of Yahoo Health, it's my job to find solutions to the food and fitness challenges that my readers struggle with—and to help them navigate the complex world of wellness.

I know that the advice in this book will help you look and feel 20 pounds younger, but that's not my only goal. My greatest aspiration is to help you find healing—for your body and your relationship with it. You shouldn't feel guilty about eating (and enjoying) food. Nor should you criticize the body you've been given. With the help of this book, you'll learn how to cast off the "I can never have the body I want" mentality for good—and replace it with inner (and outer) confidence, satisfaction, and happiness.

Trust me, if you're feeling overwhelmed, I can relate, because I have been the woman in your mirror, the one who didn't know what her body was capable of. When I finally discovered that my body *could* be strong and powerful, and that mindfulness is the secret to gaining control over my weight and health, it felt incredible. I think you'll agree. So get ready: The new you is about to emerge. And you're going to fall madly in love with her.

XO,
Michele

10 EYE-OPENERS

Paradigm-Shifting Ideas I Hope You'll Take Away from This Book

1. **We are systemic creatures.** Every part of your body, every emotion, and every action is in some way connected to your whole being—you're not just a collection of isolated parts. That means that what you eat can (and will) influence your hormones and your emotions, and they will likewise influence what you eat. It's the same for exercise. Supplements. Cosmetics. Your environment. Everything is interconnected. Everything impacts your body. When you start thinking about your body this way, you can't help but make better, healthier choices. And they become easier to adopt!

2. **You can change the foods you crave.** I used to eat a crazy amount of candy, but I've learned that too much added sugar (or salt, for that matter) masks the taste of real food. The truth is, artificial "enhancement" just detracts from the natural goodness of your meal. Once I started focusing on real food—fresh fruits and vegetables, lean meats, nuts—and cutting out the processed "fake" food, my taste buds experienced an awakening.

3. **Strength training is not just for guys.** I kind of loathe cardio. There, I said it. I know it probably sounds bananas coming from a health editor. Trust me, I understand the importance of keeping my heart in shape, which is why I squeeze in just enough cardio to be responsible. But my best body-reshaping and weight-loss results have come from resistance training. There's genius in a set of dumbbells.

4. **Quinoa—for breakfast!** Damn straight! By now, we've all heard about—and maybe even tried—the exalted quinoa grain, but my team of Life Stylists has helped me realize how incredibly versatile this ancient grain is. These days, I even eat it for breakfast! And why not? It's delicious and filling. One of the few sources of complete protein (meaning it contains all of the essential amino acids) in the grain family, it's also totally unprocessed and super convenient. I often cook a big batch so I can eat it for several days in a row, mixing it with greens and veggies for

a heartier lunch salad, sometimes making it sweet with almond milk and berries, other times making it savory with a poached egg and chili flakes on top. Give it a try. Experiment with add-ins to develop your favorite recipes, just as I've done.

5. **Small changes make a big difference.** Big goals can be overwhelming. I'm a big fan of small, incremental life tweaks. A while back, for example, I vowed to eat breakfast at my table, rather than scarfing down the most important meal of the day while emptying my dishwasher. I eat healthier. I eat slower. I enjoy the food more (and eat less). What tiny change can you make today that will pay off big-time down the road? You'll find lots of ideas in the pages that follow.

6. **Meditation won't take away your edge.** I used to think that meditation would dull my drive, make me less of a go-getter at work. But once I started practicing Transcendental Meditation, I realized that the exact opposite was true: Taking 20 minutes twice a day to refocus sharpens my senses and helps me react less emotionally to stress. In Chapter 4, you'll learn some easy ways to use mindfulness (and even try some beginner meditation) to gain control over every part of your life.

7. **Cooking is fun!** Growing up, I had zero interest in learning how to cook. I was quite content to eat a bowl of cereal for dinner or order takeout. Even when I first moved to New York City after college, I would happily eat Italian for breakfast, Greek for lunch, and Thai for dinner. Who needed to waste time hovering over a stove? I thought the idea of cooking was antifeminist. Boy was I wrong. Fast-forward to today, and cooking is one of my greatest passions. What changed? I've developed a deep appreciation for good food and have realized that the best way to ensure that I'm eating fresh, high-quality ingredients—while still enjoying what's on my plate—is to prepare it myself. That's not to say that I don't enjoy eating out. I do. I just do it less frequently than I did before.

8. **Wearing sunscreen is _the_ best thing you can do for your skin.** You simply can't expect to fry your face in the sun and still look young—especially once you hit your forties, when your skin starts to reflect all of the unwise choices you made in your twenties and thirties. That's why I apply sunscreen daily. But it has to be the right kind. Check out Chapter 12 for my recommendations.

9. **Rest—not just sleep—is critical.** Everybody who has ever opened an issue of *Women's Health* or clicked into Yahoo Health knows that poor sleep is linked to practically every health woe you can imagine. But it took me a while to realize that rest—just relaxing and unplugging for a while, not necessarily sleeping—is equally critical. I'm a typical type A personality: I rarely go totally off the grid (even on vacation), I live in one of the biggest cities in the world, I have a high-pressure job, and I thrive under pressure. All of that is to say that I'm not very good at resting, but I've learned to take the occasional breather, because relaxation is so inextricably tied to health and happiness. You'll learn to do this from our masters of bliss in Chapter 3.

10. **Oils are secret antiagers.** I'm not talking about the type you put on your food (although olive oil *is* life-affirming stuff). I mean the stuff you put on your skin. Try virgin coconut oil as an all-over moisturizer; it's amazing. And argan oil is fantastic for your face; it totally gives you the glow! And, well, why not try a bit of olive oil on your lips?

{You—In Control}

Stop the Age Accelerators

20 Pounds Younger isn't a diet plan, although good nutrition is part of it. It's a series of steps to help you gain control over those runaway trains that can accelerate aging no matter how young you are, including:

> mindless eating and weight gain

> stress (both oxidative and mental)

> high blood sugar

> loss of skeletal muscle and bone density

> the sun and other skin enemies

You can control each one of these factors. Really, you can! And doing so will lead to a weight loss of 10, 20, 30, or even more pounds and a leaner, stronger body; greater energy; improved mood; a sharper mind; and more. Each tiny bit of progress you make in each category helps you in all other areas to build a powerful force against the inward and outward signs of aging. You'll feel them working during the first week. Let's take a quick look at the five key Age Accelerators affecting women and how you will defeat them.

AGE ACCELERATOR #1: *Mindless Eating and Weight Gain*

Never underestimate the seductive power of a bag of salty chips or chocolate-covered pretzels. There are a zillion diets out there, and every one of them will fail unless you can control mindless or emotional overeating and until you can stare down a can of Pringles and use the power of your mind to keep your hand from reaching inside. Portion control, smarter choices, calorie crunching, high protein, grapefruit pectin, *whatever*—any diet technique you choose can get decent results if you understand that you have ultimate control over what you put into your mouth. No M&M's cartoon character is holding a gun to your head and saying, "Eat, or else!"

HOW YOU'LL CONTROL IT: By slowing down and engaging your mind before you munch. In Chapter 5, you'll learn various simple techniques to put the breaks on emotional eating and master the secret to enjoying your food more without feeling deprived. You can do this!

AGE ACCELERATOR #2: *Stress*

Everyone is all too familiar with stress. And unfortunately, we know from both anecdotal and scientific evidence that many owners of XX chromosomes tend to soothe stress with food. But here's the double whammy: A lot of those go-to soothing foods—high-calorie refined carbohydrates (pasta and baked goods), sugars (ice cream and alcohol), and processed meats— trigger another type of stress called oxidative stress. Free radicals (you've heard of them) are by-products of your mitochondria's processing of food energy and oxygen, and they damage cells and tissues. Oxidation is what happens to a slice of apple that browns when it's left on the counter. Similar "rusting" occurs in your body and especially in your skin. Cocktails, wine, beer? They increase levels of inflammatory molecules called cytokines, which are linked to this oxidative stress.

HOW YOU'LL CONTROL IT: Fortunately, the same strategies that will control your weight will ease both mental stress and the oxidative kind: Practicing mindfulness, eating more healthfully, and exercising the smart woman's way (which you'll learn from this book) will all help. We also suggest that you refrain from drinking alcohol for at least the first 4 weeks of the 20 Pounds Younger program. Doing so will significantly speed up weight loss and the reduction of both types of stress.

AGE ACCELERATOR #3: *High Blood Sugar and Diabetes*

Diabetes is a dangerous disease affecting about 29 million Americans. It is estimated that 86 million Americans over age 20 have the precursor to type 2 diabetes (called prediabetes), which is marked by elevated blood sugar. The majority don't know they have the problem. Prediabetes and type 2 diabetes are caused by a diet high in sugary foods and beverages and other fast-burning carbohydrates that overload your bloodstream with more glucose (your body's fuel) than the hormone insulin can usher into your muscle cells. Diabetes occurs when your body becomes resistant to insulin or your pancreas stops producing enough.

Glycation is a result of chronic high blood sugar, too. Your red blood cells get coated—or glycated—like strawberries dipped in sugar, and they start to stick together. When your tissues become loaded with glycated cells, they produce substances that further damage cells and lead to many of the symptoms of aging, including diabetes, Alzheimer's, cataracts, cardiovascular problems—even wrinkles! They call these substances advanced glycation end products or, aptly, AGEs.

HOW YOU'LL CONTROL IT: Well, one way to beat the AGEs is to find a healthier substitute for the already sugary cereal that you sprinkle sugar on every morning. Nix your soda habit. Replace doughnuts with a bowl of yogurt topped with sunflower seeds or slivered almonds. Oh, there are many, many, many easy ways to fight glycation, and you'll learn to practice them every day using our nutrition program, found in Chapter 8.

AGE ACCELERATOR #4: *Muscle and Bone Loss*

Starting at about age 30, both women and men start naturally losing muscle mass. You might not think that news is as terrible for you as it is for your buff boyfriend, but trust me, it's not good. Here's why: Studies show that for every pound of muscle you lose, you typically gain a pound of fat. Now, muscle doesn't *become* fat, it just shrinks and is replaced by fat. And because fat is less metabolically active than muscle (it burns fewer calories by simply existing), the more fat you have, the more fat you'll store in the future.

HOW YOU'LL CONTROL IT: You'll build lean muscle with weight-bearing resistance exercises to fight the natural shrinkage that scientists call *sarcopenia*. Your 3-day strength-training program, custom-made for women by trainer Holly Perkins, is easy enough for beginners and can be made more challenging as you build strength (see Chapter 10). Free bonus benefit: Your bones will become more dense and strong because weight lifting is the best way to spur new bone growth.

AGE ACCELERATOR #5: *The Sun and Other Skin Enemies*

Your skin is your armor, your body's first line of defense against the slings and barbs of daily life. Its main nemesis is easy to spot high in the sky on a summer day—it's the giver of life, and UVB rays. You know that overexposure to the sun damages cells, chips away at the structure of collagen, and causes wrinkles. You can see and feel the hot, red skin caused by a day in the sun. But there's another, more insidious age accelerator that you can't see: The free-radical assault of oxidative stress caused by a poor diet can cause blotchy pigmentation and break down the structural framework of the skin, triggering wrinkles and saggy bags just as easily as a tanning salon. Some of that oxidative stress does come from UV radiation, but much is derived internally by way of metabolic reactions from the food choices you make, and especially glycation from elevated blood sugar. (See Age Accelerators #3 and #4.)

HOW YOU'LL CONTROL IT: You'll adopt the motto of police forces throughout the world: Protect and serve. First, you'll protect your skin by blocking the UV onslaught with the right sunscreens and moisturizers, then you'll learn about and eat the foods that provide nutrients that shield against free-radical damage and reduce the occurrence of AGEs. And then, aah, you'll pamper. The skin-care and beauty regimens in Chapters 12 and 13 will show you dozens of ways to mask structural glitches and accentuate your finest features for the world to see.

Meet the
20 POUNDS
YOUNGER
Life Stylists

These are the incredible women behind the self-improvement, self-empowerment advice in *20 Pounds Younger*.

Gabrielle Bernstein

Motivational speaker, spiritual teacher, and certified Kundalini yoga instructor

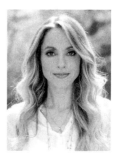

Gabrielle Bernstein has been meditating since she was a little girl—her mother taught her how—and she hasn't missed a day in the past decade. She credits the quiet time with helping her tap into her life's purpose: serving others. The *New York Times* bestselling author of *Miracles Now,* Bernstein was named "a new role model" by the *New York Times.* She is the founder of HerFuture.com, a social networking site for women to inspire, empower, and connect with one another. Find her at gabbyb.tv.

{YOGA}

Kathryn Budig

Yoga teacher on YogaGlo.com and author of
The Women's Health Big Book of Yoga

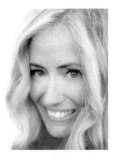

In her early twenties, Kathryn Budig moved to
Los Angeles to pursue acting, while teaching yoga on
the side. Her temporary job became a permanent one,
thanks to the enlightening lesson she learned from
yoga: Self-acceptance is the key to strength and beauty. Budig is a frequent contributor to *Women's Health,* Huffington Post, and *Yoga Journal.* She's the source
of the yoga sequences starting on page 169. Find her at KathrynBudig.com.

{DERMATOLOGY}

Francesca J. Fusco, MD

*Assistant clinical professor of dermatology at the Icahn
School of Medicine at Mount Sinai Hospital*

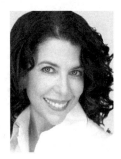

Francesca Fusco, MD, believes that combating aging
early in life with basic, noninvasive treatments—like
the skin-care regimen in this book—can allow your
complexion to retain a youthful glow and mature with
natural beauty. A member of the American Chemical Society (she even formu-
lates custom skin-care potions for some patients), Dr. Fusco has been practicing dermatology in New York City since 1990 and is an assistant clinical
professor of dermatology at the Icahn School of Medicine at Mount Sinai Hospital. She's also a *Women's Health* advisory board member for dermatology and
has been featured in the *New York Times, Allure, Elle,* and *InStyle.* Find her at
wexlerdermatology.com/meet-our-experts/francesca-fusco.

{NUTRITION}

Keri Glassman, MS, RD

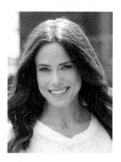

Founder and president of Keri Glassman, Nutritious Life, and The Nutrition School, a 12-week online educational program for pursuing a career as a nutritionist in New York City

Keri Glassman was destined to become a nutritionist: She recalls telling a friend in the seventh grade, "I'm craving almonds, my body must need vitamin E." Today she owns a nutrition practice and wellness brand, Nutritious Life. She also founded The Nutrition School, a program for people wanting to pursue a career in nutrition, and is the author of *The New You and Improved Diet, The O2 Diet,* and *Slim Calm Sexy Diet,* as well as a contributor to and advisory board member at *Women's Health.* "The key to successful dieting—and it's hard to do—is listening to your body telling you that it's satisfied," she says. Find her at nutritiouslife.com.

{STRENGTH TRAINING}

Holly Perkins, CSCS

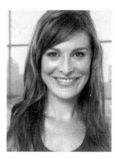

Strength training expert, founder of Women's Strength Nation, author of Women's Health Lift to Get Lean *(on sale April 2015), and owner of Holly Perkins Fitness in Los Angeles, California*

Like a lot of women, Holly Perkins shunned weight lifting and spent all of her workout time doing cardio. Frustrated by her inability to lose weight, she turned to strength training—that's right, pumping iron!—and it totally changed her life. Now she's a certified strength and conditioning specialist who teaches the benefits of resistance training with barbells, dumbbells, and machines. Her vision: to see just as many women as men in weight rooms—and to help them equal men in lifting technique and strength. In addition to being a contributing writer for *Women's Health, Prevention,* and other magazines, Perkins is the Fitness Ambassador to New Balance and author of *Women's Health Lift to Get Lean.* Find her at hollyperkins.com.

{INTERNAL MEDICINE}

Keri Peterson, MD

Internal medicine specialist at Lenox Hill Hospital, New York City

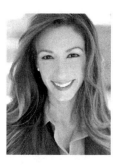

Keri Peterson, MD, considers practicing medicine less of a career and more of a life path. As she puts it, "I was premed in nursery school—I wanted to be a doctor out of the womb." Dr. Peterson considers herself much more than a primary-care physician to the people she cares for—she's a psychologist, nutritionist, and friend all rolled into one, with the ultimate goal of helping patients age with the best quality of life possible. In addition to writing a column for *Women's Health* and frequently appearing on the magazine's behalf as an expert on TV programs such as the *Today* show, she also serves as a medical advisor to HealthiNation.com. Find her at kerimd.com.

{STRUCTURAL INTEGRATION THERAPY}

Lauren Roxburgh, BCSI, CPI, CPT

Fascia and foam-rolling expert, board-certified structural integrator, certified Pilates instructor, and personal trainer

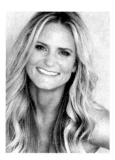

Lauren Roxburgh is considered one of the country's premier fascia and fitness experts. Dubbed the "Body Whisperer" by her loyal client following, which includes numerous celebrities and professional athletes, Roxburgh has studied health and wellness and has a degree in nutrition and exercise science as well as certifications in Pilates and pre- and postnatal yoga, anatomy, nutrition, and massage. She is a structural integration practitioner (aka a fascia expert). After studying the body, mind, and spirit for more than 20 years, Roxburgh created her signature technique, called Body Breakthru—a body-transforming, muscular-sculpting, stress-releasing fascial remodeling technique that utilizes her secret weapon, the foam roller. Visit her at laurenroxburgh.com.

{HORMONAL HEALTH}

Alisa Vitti, HHC

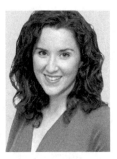

Integrative nutritionist, holistic health counselor, hormone expert, founder of FLOliving.com and author of WomanCode

Alisa Vitti is an integrative nutritionist who teaches women how to use their hormonal and neurochemical patterns to create extraordinary lives. She is the bestselling author of *Woman-Code* and the founder of FLOliving.com, a venture backed virtual health center that supports women's hormonal and reproductive health. A graduate of Johns Hopkins University and the Institute for Integrative Nutrition, she is the creator of the WomanCode System, an online learning and support program for women in their 20s, 30s, and 40s based on her functional nutritional protocol. Vitti has contributed to *The Dr. Oz Show,* CBS, Fox, *Shape*, the Huffington Post, and her own Web series on Lifetime. Her popular talk has been watched by nearly a half million people. Vitti is a sought-after speaker and has presented at Talks@Google, Summit Series Outside, Hay House, SHE Summit, and TEDx. Find her at FLOliving.com.

CHAPTER 1

What You'll Gain by Losing/

The Power of Control is Within You and the Benefits Come Fast

> How you treat *yourself* sets the standard
> for how others will treat you.
>
> – STEVE MARABOLI, MOTIVATIONAL SPEAKER

TWENTY POUNDS! THAT'S A SIGNIFICANT AMOUNT OF WEIGHT. And there's a huge cross section of women who want and need to lose 20 pounds to be healthier. But that doesn't mean 20 is for everyone. Some of you will want to lose more. Some will need to lose less for good health. We chose 20 because it's an amount of weight loss that typically improves many life functions.

Consider this: If you currently weigh 166 pounds—the average size of an American woman, according to the Centers for Disease Control and Prevention—shedding 20 pounds means losing 12 percent of your body weight. Clinical research shows that this percentage of weight reduction is where your body really starts to respond in amazing, positive ways. "The 5 to 10 percent mark is usually where the health benefits start to come in—when people start to see clinically meaningful changes in blood pressure and cholesterol," says Katie Rickel, PhD, a clinical psychologist and weight-loss expert who works at a weight-management facility in Durham, North Carolina.

1

A 20-pound drop is a visual event, too. It's when you start to turn heads and when it's obvious that you've made a "Wow!"-worthy lifestyle change. It just so happens that dropping 20 pounds is also the point at which you start feeling really good about yourself, emotionally strong and confident. In a study in the journal *Obesity*, overweight women said they'd be satisfied if they shed 15 to 20 pounds—a large enough loss to make them feel accomplished and proud. "This is a doable goal for most people who have substantial weight to lose," says Dr. Rickel.

And get this: Scientists call 20 pounds "modest" weight loss. But perhaps they're just being, well, modest, because the benefits can be totally life changing. For most women, losing 20 pounds doesn't just improve their cardiovascular health, cholesterol profile, blood sugar levels, and other biomarkers, it can actually make them look and feel years younger, feel more energetic, and experience an increased desire for sex. Pique your interest, maybe? Here's a short list of other benefits to motivate you to take up the *20 Pounds Younger* challenge today.

YOU'LL SLEEP BETTER

The soundness of your shut-eye depends on more than the quality of your mattress. In a recent study from Sweden, overweight people who dropped 14 percent of their body weight woke up fewer times during the night and spent more time actually sleeping, not just restlessly lying awake, counting mini meatballs in bed. The slimmed-down sleepers also began spending a larger portion of each night in deep sleep, a phase that's important for overall well-being, metabolism, and healthy blood pressure, the scientists say. As a result, they felt less sleepy during the day, which is significant because research shows that when we're weary, we may be more likely to reach for unhealthy, easy-access foods. "I'm bushed. Time for a candy bar!"

One of the first places skimping on sleep shows up is on facial skin. Tired people look older, since their lack of energy often translates to a droopy facade. (Think Eeyore in *Winnie the Pooh*.) A 2013 Swedish study found that after just 31 hours of sleep deprivation, people appeared to have droopier lids; redder eyes; darker under-eye circles; paler skin; and more wrinkles. They even looked sadder, and we all know what kind of first impression a frown makes.

YOU'LL PROTECT YOUR HEART

Lugging around extra pounds puts undue strain on your arteries. Luckily, losing weight can reverse this threat: Obese people who shed 10 percent of their body weight through a combination of diet and exercise saw an 11 percent reduction in their systolic blood pressure (the top number) and a 7-point drop in their diastolic pressure (the bottom number), a recent study in the *Journal of the American Medical Association* found.

YOU'LL SHED DANGEROUS BELLY FAT

The same study that found that weight loss caused a reduction in blood pressure (see above) found another key result of losing roughly 20 pounds: significant loss of deep abdominal fat. Visceral fat, the technical name for the stuff that cozies up to your internal organs, is surprisingly responsive to lifestyle changes, say Harvard scientists. This is good news because visceral fat is not just unsightly: It's also the kind of fat most strongly associated with a heightened risk of type 2 diabetes and heart disease, the study authors say.

The best way to target belly fat? Add physical activity to your weight-loss plan from the get-go. In the study, people who started exercising at the same time they began dieting lost more lard from around their midsections than those who put off exercising for 6 months. That suggests that physical activity in combination with diet can specifically target that troublesome fat that complements no swimsuit.

WORKING OUT WILL BE EASIER

Imagine taking a walk around the block with a big sack of dog chow strapped to your back. That'd be pretty uncomfortable (though it would make you very popular with the neighborhood puppies). Well, the same goes for carrying around extra weight: "If you have 20 pounds of extra fat, it's like wearing a 20-pound weight vest while doing jumping jacks," says Wayne Westcott, PhD, an instructor of exercise science at Quincy College. "That puts a lot more stress on your muscles, joints, and cardiovascular system. The lower your weight, the easier exercise will be." As will walking up stairs, getting out of Lotus pose in yoga, and catching speedy toddlers.

YOU'LL GIVE YOUR CAREER A BOOST

The unfortunate truth about being overweight: You're at risk of being discriminated against in the workplace. In a 2012 study, for example, German researchers found that nearly half of human resource professionals opted to disqualify obese female job candidates when presented with a group of potential hires. The sad truth is thin people are more likely to be hired and out-earn their heavier counterparts by almost $19,000 per year, according to research in the *Journal of Applied Psychology.*

YOU'LL FEEL MORE CONFIDENT

When you don't love the skin you're in, that self-loathing feeling can carry over to every aspect of your life, including your career, love life, and friendships. Case in point: In a 2010 study in the *Journal of Health Psychology*, overweight women admitted to avoiding social gatherings—or trying to go unnoticed when they did leave the house. They felt that their size was a central part of their identity—that they were "big" and therefore "unattractive." What happened after these women lost at least 10 percent of their body weight, or roughly 20 pounds? They felt liberated—less socially reserved—and like their body shape didn't define them. Makes sense, no? When you feel secure in your body, do you waste time scrutinizing your muffin top? No. You're too busy having fun!

YOUR BRAIN WILL ACT YOUNGER

As your waist gets larger, your brain's capacity may shrink. Research suggests that obesity can impair your episodic memory, the part of your brain that helps you recall past events in your life (such as your first date). Luckily, recent Swedish research suggests that losing weight may undo this damage. The researchers tested overweight women's episodic memory before and after they slimmed down, and they found that their recall improved (and became more efficient) after they dropped an average of 18 pounds. Genius!

YOU'LL HAVE MORE ENERGY

Extra weight drags you down physically and mentally. But even losing just 5 pounds can boost your energy and zest for life, according to a study in the journal *Health Psychology*. Imagine how amazing you'll feel after dropping 20! Bonus: The dieters in the study also felt less depressed and anxious after slimming down. Your mental booster shot is just a few pages away.

YOUR POSTURE WILL IMPROVE

When lugging around extra weight, it can be tough to stand tall. According to a 2010 Italian study, obesity may encourage you to tilt your pelvis forward (in a stance similar to the one heavily pregnant women adopt), predisposing you to lower back pain. Losing 20 pounds (or less) will help you stand upright again, and that will make it appear that you've lost even more weight than you have! "Good posture makes you look younger, thinner, and taller," says Rebecca Gorrell, a former movement therapist at Canyon Ranch spa. "Other people will see you as more energetic and relaxed."

YOUR SEX LIFE WILL SIZZLE

If you feel better about your body, you won't be worrying as much about your stomach jiggling while doing the reverse cowgirl with your guy—and less distraction almost always equals more pleasure and more sex! After losing 13.5 percent of their body weight, overweight women reported having sex twice as often as before—and they felt more aroused, lubricated, and satisfied while doing so, according to a 2013 study in the *Journal of Sexual Medicine*.

INSTANT AGE ERASER
A Brief Nap

Research shows that short naps decrease fatigue, improve alertness and cognitive performance, and leave you looking refreshed. And hey, you deserve to take five. Speaking of time, the optimum amount of shut-eye is 5 to 15 minutes. Set an alarm. Snoozing for more than 30 can leave you groggy.

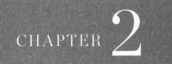

CHAPTER 2

Why We Eat the Way We Do/

Understanding the Emotions That Drive You To Food Will Help You Stop Swallowing Your Feelings

> Gluttony is an *emotional* escape, a sign something is eating *us*.
>
> —PETER DE VRIES, FORMER ESSAYIST FOR THE *NEW YORKER*

EATING IS RARELY JUST ABOUT, WELL, EATING. Food plays many roles in our lives, and we eat for many, many different reasons unrelated to the biological need for sustenance—331 reasons, to be exact, according to a German study in the journal *Appetite*. We eat when we're sad or stressed. We eat when we're celebrating. We eat because our friends are eating. We eat because the jelly beans are within arm's reach.

Those German researchers sorted the reasons into 15 core motives. Check 'em out; you'll recognize many of your own drivers for diving in that have nothing to do with being hungry. Getting to know them is one key to mastering mindful eating, which is the key to the 20 Pounds Younger eating plan.

1. **Liking:** I eat this food because it tastes good.*
2. **Habit:** This is something I'm accustomed to eating regularly.

3.   **Need and hunger:** I am hungry or need an energy boost.*

4.   **Health:** I'm trying to maintain a balanced diet or stay in shape, and this food will fulfill my nutritional needs.*

5.   **Convenience:** This food is quick or easy to prepare, convenient, or readily available.

6.   **Pleasure:** I want to indulge or reward myself. This food puts me in a good mood.*

7.   **Tradition:** My family always eats this food on this holiday. I always snack on this food during this activity.*

8.   **Natural concerns:** This food is organic, fair trade, environmentally friendly, or natural.*

9.   **Sociability:** It's pleasant to eat with others. Eating makes social gatherings more enjoyable or comfortable.*

10. **Price:** This item is inexpensive, on sale, free, or I've already purchased it.

11. **Visual appeal:** The package is appealing, the food is nicely presented, or I recognize this item from advertisements.*

12. **Weight control:** This food is low in fat or calories, and I'm trying to lose weight.*

13. **Emotional regulation:** I'm sad, frustrated, lonely, bored, or stressed, and this food cheers me up.*

14. **Social norms:** It would be impolite not to eat this—I wouldn't want to disappoint.

15. **Social image:** This food is trendy right now and reinforces the image I want to portray.

* This reason for eating was more often cited by women than men.

As you can see, sitting down for a meal can be as complicated as your high school love life. Note that the researchers found that women are especially prone to eating for emotional reasons, and that's the kind of feasting that often leads to weight gain.

Researchers observing kids eating ice cream have found that most of them stop eating when they feel full, even though there's still ice cream left in the bowl. Not so for adults. Researchers say that we've been conditioned over the years by emotional and social cues to keep shoveling it in. We think, "Gosh, I love this so much that I need to eat every bite to maximize my experience—even if by the last spoonful I'm groaning." In a recent survey of more than 1,300 psychologists, 43 percent cited emotional eating as a barrier to weight loss. "[We] have a bad day and self-medicate with food," says Linda Spangle, RN, MA, a Denver-based weight-loss coach. "Emotional eating is the number-one reason most diets fail."

As an extreme example, binge eating—which is now classified as a full-on eating disorder—is characterized by a total loss of control while eating and a tendency to eat a huge volume of food in response to feelings, rather than actual physical hunger. Although most of us don't qualify as binge eaters, the psychological underpinnings of the disorder can show up in anybody—even someone who isn't uncontrollably scarfing down egregious amounts of food on a regular basis.

"[It's] absolutely not limited to going home and eating your whole pantry," says Heather Niemeier, PhD, an associate professor of psychology at the University of Wisconsin–Whitewater. "It's not a disorder. It's something that a lot of us do." Some researchers have even called emotional eating an "invisible plague," since so many of us do it but so few talk about it.

So where do things go wrong? The simple answer: Life happens. We experience the beauty and pleasure of food; we build memories around the joy and guilt and reward of eating. Our relationship with food becomes about much more than simply fueling our bodies. It gets complex—and often more tumultuous than any romantic entanglement. Yes, boyfriends can cause you to go a little crazy, but you can always walk away from those relationships. You and food, on the other hand, are stuck together for life. This is one of your most important relationships; it pays to take some time to get it right.

The Origins of Comfort Foods

Our nation's epidemic of emotional overeating boils down to the food and feeling connections that our brains are so adept at making, which Dr. Rickel says we start to form even in infancy. "When we're babies and we cry, what do our caretakers do?" she asks. "They give us a bottle or breast-feed us. So we instantly learn: 'I cry, I get food, the world is okay again.'" Later, milk is replaced by milk shakes—or some other food we associate with comfort.

Why can't we just crave fruits and veggies, since they are, after all, what our bodies need most? It's because the foods we consider comforting

4 SNEAKY OVEREATING TRIGGERS

1. Commercials for Yummy-Looking Food

A 2011 study in the *Journal of Consumer Policy* found that female emotional eaters tend to be highly influenced by ads for indulgent foods—so much so that a single commercial was capable of sending them into a cycle of repetitive thoughts about the food.

2. There's Food Left on Your Plate

If you're a lifetime member of the Clean Plate Club, you probably overwhelmed your body's "I'm full!" signals a long time ago by consistently scraping up every crumb because, as your dad told you, "Children are starving in China." You no longer do other things that Mom and Dad demanded, so why do this one? Break the cycle by getting into the habit of leaving something on your plate at every meal.

3. You Drive By a Favorite Restaurant

Lesley Lutes, PhD, an associate professor of psychology at East Carolina University, recalls a woman in one of her weight-loss studies who vowed to eat a healthy breakfast at home, yet couldn't seem to break her morning date with Krispy Kreme. "One morning, she was driving to work and all of a sudden the hot doughnut sign for Krispy Kreme came on," she says. Even though the woman had already eaten a healthy breakfast, the car practically pulled itself into the drive-thru. "That hot doughnut sign was such a strong external cue to her that it was overriding her already having had breakfast," says Dr. Lutes.

4. Your Must-Watch TV Show

Are you a TV *diner*? A Harvard study examining more than 50,000 women's lifestyle habits found that obesity rates increased by 23 percent for every 2 hours of watching television, and incidences of type 2 diabetes shot up by 14 percent. It wasn't all due to the sedentary nature of their lifestyles, either: Increased munching while watching added to the mindless calorie boost.

are often the ones we associate with positive emotions through our culture and our families—for example, a snack you always ate with your grandma as a little girl may become a go-to munchie when you're stressed. The foods you ate in your dorm room after a fun night out with your girlfriends, the lunch your mom always made for you as a kid, the snacks you stowed away at summer camp—all of these can carry strong emotional ties, which may compel you to seek them out in times of stress, celebration, or sadness.

Some of the reasons we are attracted to certain foods are hardwired. A brain-scan study conducted at the University of Oxford showed that fat's oily sensation in the mouth lights up the orbitofrontal cortex, a part of the brain that registers pleasantness. This, in turn, may drive the urge to eat more.

Load up a fatty food with sugar—think ice cream, cake, and doughnuts—

and it's a double whammy. Sugary treats elevate your levels of ghrelin, a hormone that acts as a powerful appetite stimulant and increases cravings. You may tell yourself, "Just one bite," but find that the more you eat, the more you want. It's your brain's reward system at play: "The brain responds to both sugar and fat by releasing [feel-good brain chemicals called] endorphins," says Gary Wenk, PhD, a professor of psychology and neuroscience at Ohio State University. This is something food manufacturers are all too aware of. They've even coined a term for it: They call it the "bliss point"—the perfect balance of ingredients (often sweeteners) to make people crave a food, buy it, and keep taking just one more bite...and then another.

Why Women Fall Prey to Emotional Eating

Everyone—man or woman—eats for emotional reasons. However, studies show that females—whether they are rats or humans—tend to overeat in response to feeling stressed, lonely, nervous, or depressed, likely as a way to numb, distract, or soothe themselves, while depressed males tend to eat less.

Why was Mother Nature so unfair to us? Unfortunately, there's no single, solid explanation for why women flock to food in times of trouble, although some scientists think women are simply more responsive to food rewards than men are. "It could be biological reasons, as well as social and cultural reasons," says Jennifer Daubenmier, PhD, an assistant professor at the Osher Center for Integrative Medicine at the University of California—San Francisco.

For starters, there are those ever-annoying, ever-fluctuating female hormones, which, as any woman can attest, make you feel simultaneously moody and famished (a totally volatile combo). The midluteal phase of a woman's cycle—which occurs right before menstruation—is an especially vulnerable time for emotional eating, likely because progesterone levels and estradiol are high, according to a new study from Michigan State University.

But female hormones aren't entirely to blame (although they are a convenient scapegoat!); emotional eating may also be a way to avoid dealing with psychological stress. Eating away our feelings can be a more comfortable, safe way to deal than confronting a problem head-on.

FOOD FRENEMIES

Another step in fighting emotional eating is recognizing the impact your friends and relatives—your potential *food frenemies*—may have on your diet. In a 2012 study from Stanford University, 90 percent of women participating in a weight-loss program said they rarely or never receive support from their friends for healthy eating. Seventy-eight percent said the same about their family. A number of the dieters even reported that loved ones *sabotage* their efforts to slim down.

Suspect you have a few weight-loss saboteurs? Ann Kearney-Cooke, PhD, director of the Cincinnati Psychotherapy Institute, suggests asking yourself these four questions.

> Who are the three people I'm closest to?

> How do I eat before, after, and while I'm with them?

> Are they meeting my expectations and emotional needs? (For example, is my boyfriend there for me when I'm having a crappy day and need someone to talk to? Does he turn off the TV when I want to spend time together?)

> When these people don't meet my expectations, what can I do to deal with my stress without straying from my weight-loss plan?

You may find that you're infuriated when your mom calls during work hours, and you feel like you need an ice cream bar afterward. Or maybe you constantly feel coerced into ordering margaritas with your best friend because she'll call you a fun-killer if you don't. Once you recognize these social triggers, strategize accordingly: Screen your calls so you can call your mom back when you're free, or ask your gal pal if you can do pedicures in lieu of happy hour. They may be disappointed at first, but they'll adjust. Stress and food frenemies often coexist. The solution lies in developing the strength to take control of both.

In the next chapter, we will look more closely at how stress can trigger a feeding frenzy and explore simple ways to chill. After all, stress has a major impact on your belly, your body, and your mind, which ages more quickly under stress.

THREE TAKEAWAYS TO TRY TODAY

1. **Don't be a member of the Clean Plate Club.** Get into the habit of leaving some food on your plate at every meal.

2. **Question your motives.** Women tend to be emotional eaters. Next time you reach for a bag of chips or a doughnut, pause and ask yourself: Am I hungry, or is one of those other 14 motives for eating driving me to munch?

3. **Ask yourself the "food frenemies" questions** and develop a better response to social cues to eat.

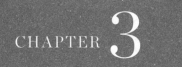

CHAPTER 3

Erasing Stress/
Time to Start Making Yourself
Priority Number One

When a woman becomes her own *best friend* life is easier.

–DIANE VON FURSTENBERG, DESIGNER

STRESS IS A FAMILIAR COMPANION TO MOST WOMEN because so much of it stems from a lack of time. You have too much on your plate, too many people asking you for too many things, and not enough time to get it all done. But there's another type of stress that's even more insidious: the stress you place on yourself when you feel you don't measure up—to your own expectations or to other people's. Either type of stress can make you more vulnerable to emotional eating or just saying, "Screw it all!"

Consider this: When the pressure mounts, 66 percent of women reach to sweet foods for relief, according to a survey in the journal *Physiology and Behavior.* When they are finished scarfing, 51 percent of them feel guilty about it.

Emotional eating is a vicious cycle: The stress you place on yourself in striving to be skinny may lead you to overeat. And when you overeat, you may think you have no self-restraint and feel weak, out of control, or disgusted with your own behavior. Talk about a double dose of stress!

This self-judgment stuff can cue a chronic deluge of the stress hormone cortisol, which also happens to be one of the most potent appetite signals we have, triggering cravings for highly sweetened, fatty, processed foods. By repeatedly stressing out and then coping by eating, people can experience neurobiological adaptations that can lead to compulsive over-eating, scientists say. Stress eating essentially becomes a reflex, so you no longer engage the problem-solving part of your brain when you're trying to cope—you just turn to the junk food.

You'll remember from the last chapter that the so-called comfort foods you crave tend to be high in fat, sugar, or both. They are soothing and make you feel good for as long as you're riding that carbohydrate high. But that feeling quickly fades (around the time of your sugar crash), and you end up feeling unhappy all over again.

Here's more crummy news: If your body pumps out stress hormones on a daily basis, they can begin to break down your immune, gastrointesti-nal, neurological, and musculoskeletal systems, says Nancy Molitor, PhD, an assistant professor of clinical psychiatry at Northwestern University. When cortisol levels surge, your glucose levels spike and this chemical tag team promotes fat storage, primarily in your belly. What's more, the over-load may lead to oxidative stress, which ages your cells more quickly.

Aren't you glad you're a woman? All of this may seem pretty bleak, but there's a way out of this mess: *20 Pounds Younger* to your rescue!

How to Defeat the Stress Monster

Gaining control over external stressors starts with two things: accepting that they'll always be there, and being confident that you can manage stress-ful feelings using an arsenal of mental and physical strategies. Controlling *self-induced stress* is a little more challenging because it requires accepting yourself and learning to love your body, but we have a plan for that, too. Let's start with some effective techniques for living effectively with chaos.

LEARN TO SAY NO. "Overcommitting reduces the time you have to tend to your own needs—like eating healthfully, sleeping an appropriate number of hours, or caring for your immediate family," says Nanette Gartrell, MD, author of *My Answer Is No—If That's Okay with You.* Not sure how to gracefully decline? "I simply cannot fit it into my schedule"—followed by an expression of gratitude—will suffice, says Dr. Gartrell.

GO TO SLEEP EARLIER. Fatigue raises cortisol levels and exacerbates anxiety and feelings of being out of control. What's too little sleep? Fewer than 7 hours. Ideally, try to get 7 or even 8. See how you feel after both durations, and from then on, try to get the right amount for you. Sleep is when your body repairs and rebuilds tissue. Cheat your body out of that essential process, and your skin will suffer. University Hospitals Case Medical Center in Cleveland found that women who slept 5 or fewer hours a night or who had poor-quality sleep due to tossing and turning had more signs of facial aging—like fine lines and uneven pigmentation—in just 1 week.

FIND YOUR BLISS. People who participated in "happiness training"—yep, that's a thing!—reported feeling less stressed after-ward, according to a 2013 study from Germany. So how'd they boost their spirits? They jotted down things that brought them joy each day, wrote someone a thank-you letter, did unexpected favors, gave people little presents, and enjoyed 10 minutes of daily silence. Pick one to try today.

SIP A CUP OF TEA. In a study from University College London, people who drank a cup of black tea before completing stressful tasks experienced a 47 percent drop in cortisol afterward, compared to just 27 percent in those who didn't drink tea.

HAVE MORE SEX. Scottish scientists found that people who got randy at least once every 2 weeks were better able to manage stressful situations, such as public speaking. Why? Possibly because orgasms trigger a relaxation response and bathe your body in endorphins and other feel-good brain chemicals.

PRESS THE ISSUE. Acupressure is a quick and effective tension releaser—it can reduce stress by up to 39 percent, according to researchers at Hong Kong Polytechnic University. For a fast chill drill, try massaging the fleshy area between your thumb and index finger for 20 to 30 seconds.

TAKE A VIDEO BREAK. At work, spend 60 seconds of every hour watching a funny video. Laughter is one of the world's best stress relievers—and it's free.

MEDITATE AT WORK. In a recent study from Australia, workers who meditated in their office chairs for just 15 minutes showed a significant decline in blood pressure. Not sure where to start? Download a guided meditation app for your smartphone, such as Smiling Mind or The Mindfulness App. Hint: Squeeze in your downtime during your lunch hour, so you can switch off your office phone—and therefore eliminate distractions—as the study participants did. For more meditation tips, see Chapter 4.

TAKE GUITAR LESSONS. Plant a garden. Refinish an end table. Mastering a new activity can reward you with a rush of feel-good dopamine, sending your brain into a relaxing state called "flow," where you totally lose track of time. This may explain why so many women find crafting to be cathartic.

HUG HIM. Turns out, love *is* a drug. Women who frequently hug their partners tend to have lower blood pressure than those in less-affectionate relationships, a study in the journal *Biological Psychology* suggests. The benefit may stem from oxytocin, the bonding hormone, which helps you *feel* calm and may dampen sympathetic nervous system activity—the fight-or-flight response—in your heart and blood vessels, says study author Kathleen Light, PhD.

HEAD OUTSIDE. People who live near green spaces—parks or open fields, for example—experience fewer negative effects of stress than those living with a shortage of green, a Dutch study shows. Of course, not all of us are lucky enough to enjoy a park view, but you *can* carve out time for nature walks, volunteer at a community garden, or just read a book on a park bench.

GET A MASSAGE. Everyone knows that a massage eases tense muscles, but it relieves mental tension, too. One study found that just a 15-minute chair massage lowered people's cortisol levels by 24 percent. And they noticed the difference, too: Study participants reported feeling less stressed, anxious, and depressed.

TRY THE TRICKLE EFFECT. Studies show that being near water—or hearing the sound of flowing H$_2$O—can lower your heart rate and stress levels and help you feel more serene. Even just looking at water can be soothing. So set up a plug-in tabletop fountain in your living room, arrange floating candles in clear water-filled vases, or buy a desktop fish tank filled with aquatic plants. Tight on space? Even hanging photos of ocean or river scenes—heck, just changing your computer's screen saver to one with a water theme—can lend you some of water's calming effects.

CREATE A QUIET CORNER. There's a reason spas set up hushed, low-lit lounge areas. "They're designed to make you feel swaddled, to provide comfort and security," says Simon Marxer, the spa director at Miraval Resort and Spa in Tucson. Recreating this effect at home can be as simple as arranging a few plush pillows (cool green and blue are the most calming) in a dimly lit corner of your quietest room.

Learn to Be Kinder to Yourself

The quote by Diane Von Furstenberg at the beginning of this chapter is one of my favorites because it simply sums up our reward for defeating the more challenging type of stress—that which is self-induced. Again, she said: "When a woman becomes her own best friend life is easier."

All of the beat-stress tricks and techniques above are great for dealing with the external stressors that drive you bonkers, but they won't do much if your 24-7 companion isn't cutting you some slack. Ask yourself: Are you really your best friend? When was the last time you admired your thighs or went a day without berating your body or just told yourself that you're beautiful? If you're like the unfortunate majority of women, you don't appreciate your body enough—or at all. You may even treat your worst foe with more respect and kindness, and you deserve better.

In a recent study in *Personality and Social Psychology Bulletin*, researchers asked people in 26 countries to rate their dissatisfaction with their bodies; not surprisingly, women in North America—90 percent of whom were from the United States—were the most critical of their figures. "It's an endemic problem in our culture—women are self-loathing," says Judith Hanson Lasater, PhD, PT, and author of *Living Your Yoga: Finding the Spiritual in Everyday Life*. "To meet a woman who really loves her body is rare."

This is especially true among overweight women. A 2013 study in the *Journal of Human Nutrition and Dietetics* found that as a woman's BMI increases, so does her unhappiness with her body. Or is it the other way around—that dissatisfaction breeds a higher BMI? Research has also shown that normal-weight people who view themselves as fat are more likely to end up overweight. "We know that people with very poor acceptance of their bodies may actually weigh more, either because they are so anxious about their weight that it triggers overeating or because they are so anxious, they block out any awareness," says psychologist Jean Kristeller, PhD.

It's easy to justify your self-loathing with "I'd be happy if" statements, such as:

> ❯ "I'd be happy with my body if my thighs didn't touch."

> ❯ "I'd love myself if I had a flat stomach."

> ❯ "It would be a lot easier to embrace my body if I wasn't overweight."

We live in a culture that teaches women to connect with other women with this kind of fat talk even as we preach the "healthy at any size" message. "There's been a movement toward embracing different body sizes and shapes, but the 'thin ideal' is still very dominant," says Jennifer Webb, PhD, an assistant professor of health psychology at the University of North Carolina–Charlotte. "For many of us who don't measure up to that, it creates this discrepancy, which sets you up for shame—feeling like you're a failure, and then disengaging from any form of health promotion." In other words, if you can't be supermodel skinny, you may decide not to exercise or eat healthfully, period, since there's no way you can meet others' (or your own) expectations.

But the truth is, self-love doesn't mean accepting yourself on the condition that you lose 5, 10, 15, or 20 pounds. "You have to love yourself first, and then you won't overeat," asserts Dr. Lasater. Can accepting your body really translate into better eating? Yes—and research proves that you need to adjust your nude attitude, ASAP: In a 2013 study, women with high levels of self-compassion tended to eat more intuitively. These self-accepting gals gave themselves permission to nosh whenever they were hungry, rarely ate for emotional reasons, and relied on their bodies internal cues to determine when and how much to eat. Another study from the Technical University of Lisbon showed that women who worked on improving their body image lost more weight than those who didn't try to elevate their self-esteem.

The science clearly shows that being kinder to yourself really works. But, hey, I get it: Accepting your body is tough in our culture. And it's not just a matter of flipping a switch and deciding to love your thighs; it takes conscious effort. In Your Mindful Eating Workshop (see page 223), we'll walk you through several body-acceptance exercises that you will find extremely empowering. Meanwhile, start working these simple reinforcement practices into your life.

The Keys to a Better Body Image

PAY HOMAGE. Every night before you fall asleep, thank your body for something it's done for you, suggests Dr. Lasater. A few examples: "Thank you for giving me the strength to run a mile." "Thank you for being flexible enough to do crow pose." "Thank you for giving me the ability to dance with my friends." Appreciating your body for its physical abilities—rather than focusing solely on its appearance—will help you love your figure *now*.

BOOK A MASSAGE. The pleasure of a massage has a price: You have to be willing to strip down. As terrifying as getting naked in front of a stranger may sound (you will be under a sheet, though!), letting another person touch you—even if you haven't yet reached your goal weight—can help you feel more comfortable in your own skin, says Mitch Klein, a licensed massage therapist in New York City. In fact, women who received just one 50-minute massage reported a boost in body image, a recent Bridgewater State University study found. Credit the surge of endorphins, which may teach you to associate your body with pleasure, instead of distress, the scientists say.

PRACTICE YOGA. Doing yoga can help you appreciate your body's amazing capabilities. "Yoga means unity—it's really about connecting all of the different parts of your body with your mind and spirit," says Rachel Allyn, PhD, a psychologist and yoga instructor in Minneapolis. "That's really different from the way most of us compartmentalize and objectify different parts of our bodies—as in, 'I hate my butt,' or 'I've never really liked my shape.'" In one study, women who could more accurately count their heartbeats objectified themselves less, suggesting that tuning in to the way your body works can help you dwell less on its appearance.

EXPAND YOUR DEFINITION OF EXERCISE. If joining a gym intimidates you—or you just don't enjoy exercising in that setting—find something you can love, whether that means exercising in your living room, jogging with a girlfriend, or signing up for a hiking club. If you can exercise without feeling self-conscious, you're more likely to keep at it—and your self-image will get healthier along with your body.

NEVER AIM FOR PERFECT. That will guarantee failure almost every time. Be the best you can be, but acknowledge that you will make mistakes—and then know which slipups to let go of.

ACCEPT YOUR NOT-SO-KIND THOUGHTS—BUT DON'T BELIEVE THEM. In a later chapter, you'll learn to accept—and sit with—food cravings, rather than trying to distract yourself from the call of the cookie jar. You can apply this same meditative approach to intrusive thoughts about your body. You have to come to terms with the negative self-talk. That may sound simple enough, but the truth is, it's often easier to avoid acknowledging your internal critic, because doing otherwise may require facing some pretty crappy beliefs about yourself. Instead of pushing "I'm fat" or "I can't stick to an exercise program" thoughts aside, allow them to surface—but refuse to buy into them.

SPEAK THE (BODY) LANGUAGE. Whenever you hunch your shoulders, cross your arms over your chest, or stare at the floor, you announce your self-consciousness, says body-language expert Lillian Glass, PhD. According to a study in the *European Journal of Social Psychology,* good posture is linked with higher levels of self-confidence. So try a "fake-it-till-you-make-it" experiment: Walk upright, as if a string is pulling you up from the top of your head. When you talk to someone, squeeze your butt muscles to straighten your spine, and stand with your feet a foot apart, toes pointing at the person you're facing. Smile, and don't be afraid to use your hands when you talk. This kind of openness makes you seem more secure.

ACTIVELY PURSUE SELF-ACCEPTANCE. Deciding that you're cool—even happy—with your body isn't enough. "Acceptance

FIT TIP:
Avoid Reflecting

Next time you catch yourself peering into a mirror, smile and move on. Researchers say that frequent body checking in front of the mirror for perceived flaws reinforces a negative body image.

isn't something we achieve," says Dr. Webb. "It's a value we continuously engage with, sometimes several times a day. It's about how you treat yourself." In other words, this isn't just an attitude you adopt—you have to actively show yourself kindness, in ways consistent with your goals. "One of the biggest misconceptions is that self-compassion is a vehicle for self-indulgence—that you're going to go on an eating binge and be okay with it," she says. What it actually looks like: Instead of berating yourself when you slip up, you acknowledge the mishap, choose to be in control the next moment, and continue plugging away at your goal.

REFUSE TO WALLOW. "Getting overly wrapped up in negative thought is often the doorway to self-pity—when we're thinking we're alone in our pain and suffering," says Dr. Webb. So sometimes, the kind thing to do is to kick yourself in the butt and realize that you don't have it so bad. "Intentionally recognize that you are not alone in this—that there are others experiencing similar pain," she says. "That actually helps us snap out of self-pity." Consider taking a trip to the beach or gym to check out other ladies. "Plenty of people with imperfections far worse than yours are out there flaunting it," says psychologist Barbara Keesling, PhD.

TAKE OWNERSHIP OF YOUR GOALS. If you view exercise as torture or eating vegetables as punishment, take a trip back in time: When you were a kid, did your parents force you to eat spinach? Did an ex-boyfriend say you'd be sexier if you exercised? Did your gym teacher embarrass you because you couldn't loop the track? These kinds of negative experiences can make exercise and health seem like someone else's goal—not something you've chosen to do for yourself, says Dr. Webb. So figure out why *you* want to shape up, whether it's to boost your energy, increase your sexual confidence, or just fit into your clothes better. Then keep those goals in mind whenever it's time to make a healthy choice. Suddenly, working out or eating right will feel like your idea. That's incredibly motivating.

THREE TAKEAWAYS TO TRY TODAY

1. **Say no to someone who asks you for your time or your help.** Do it once a day if you're one of those "pleasers" who can never say no. The practice will be empowering, and you'll find that you have more time for yourself.

2. **Do something nice for yourself,** like making a cup of good tea, taking a walk, or looking into the mirror, smiling, and saying "You're a damn good person—and good-looking, too."

3. **Stand and walk upright, as if there were a string attached to the top of your head and a giant pulling on it.** Good posture is linked with higher self-confidence, and it will also make you look younger and more energetic.

INSTANT AGE ERASER

Green Juice

Drinking a glass of juice is a whole lot easier than eating 5 pounds of leafy greens in a sitting. Juicing organic raw vegetables like kale, spinach, and other greens removes the fiber so the vitamins and antioxidants are more quickly absorbed into your bloodstream. By the way, the aforementioned veggies are high in polyphenols and carotenoids, two antioxidants that have been shown to protect your skin from sun damage. Drink up!

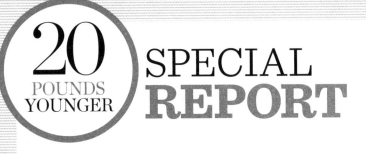
How Hormones Eff Up Your Diet

HORMONES ARE SUPERIMPORTANT CHEMICAL messengers that travel throughout your body triggering your organs to perform key functions. They affect every part of you, 24-7. They make things happen—sometimes not in the most welcome ways. Take the best known of these, the Big E. Estrogen is the Godzilla of your hormones, wreaking havoc by fueling mood swings, a raging appetite, acne, and spur-of-the-moment shopping trips—and that's just for starters. You know it well. Although it's critical, that primary female hormone is just one chemical in a crowd of hormones—including leptin, ghrelin, and insulin, among others—that can, at any given moment, wield enormous influence over how you feel and what you do. But don't worry—they can all be tamed. And that's the focus of this special report.

"When your hormones are in balance, everything about you, from the inside out, functions and looks its best," says Life Stylist Alisa Vitti, an integrative nutritionist, holistic health counselor, hormone expert, founder of FLOliving.com, and author of *WomanCode*. "When they are out of balance, however, your body begins to prematurely age hormonally, causing you to retain weight and feel sluggish." The good news is you can adjust your diet to achieve perfect balance and prolong your youth. Here are some practical nutrition tips that will go a long way toward helping you become a more successful mindful eater.

Ghrelin: The "I'm Hungry" Hormone

"Ghrelin" sounds like "gremlin"—and it's an apt comparison because it can screw with your best dieting intentions. Also known as the hunger hormone, this chemical, which is mainly produced in your stomach, awakens your appetite. It's like someone ringing the dinner bell with a buffalo wing drumstick drenched in blue cheese—it gets your attention. When your stomach is empty or you're restricting calories, ghrelin travels from cells in your stomach to your brain, where it triggers feelings of hunger. Once you eat, your levels of ghrelin tend to drop.

BALANCE IT OUT: Feeling famished? Eat something, but not *everything*. Here's where mindful eating comes into play. Certain foods tame the ghrelin beast better than others. For example, lean protein and complex carbohydrates are better at suppressing the hormone than fat is, so have sliced turkey breast or Greek yogurt to take the edge off. Eat "clean" by having a salad or cut-up vegetables. Whatever you do, when you recognize the hungry hormone's siren call, stay away from sugar-laden foods such as ice cream, cake, and doughnuts. These fast-burning carbs tend to increase ghrelin levels—and once you awaken the appetite stimulator, you'll have trouble stopping at just one bite.

Don't have any carrots in your pocket? Even thinking about healthy foods can reduce ghrelin's power. In a Yale University study, people who anticipated drinking a sensible milk shake experienced a lower spike of ghrelin than those who dreamed of a thick chocolate shake with whipped cream, a cherry, and a side of fries. So, think clean. The scientists involved in the study suggest that the "psychological mindset of sensibility" might actually dampen the effect of the hunger hormone.

Leptin: The "I'm Satisfied" Hormone

When the hormone leptin is high, you feel full and satisfied and you can focus on important tasks—returning phone calls, booking that vacation flight, sex!—instead of just thinking, "How can I get my hands on some nachos?" So how do you keep this helpful hormone pumping? Keeping your weight at a healthy level will help immensely. Research has shown that excess body fat can cause a condition known as *leptin resistance*, which means that your brain no longer responds to the hormone, even though your body contains elevated amounts of it. One explanation: As fat cells crank out inflammatory chemicals that block the appetite-suppressing effect of leptin, your body begins to think it's starving. Obviously, that's not really the case, but to compensate, your metabolism slows down and your brain bombards you with constant hunger signals.

BALANCE IT OUT: Exercising regularly and eating clean, healthy foods are two good ways to increase leptin in your body. Try this hormone-stabilizing trick: Eat 1 cup of vegetables before 10 a.m. every day. (Hint: Fold them into an omelet.) Endocrinologist Scott Isaacs, MD, has found that people who do this tend to be less hungry later in the day. Vegetables are packed with satiating fiber, as well as vitamins and anti-oxidants that have been shown to reduce the inflammation that interferes with leptin, which in turn helps increase fat burning and combat cravings.

Insulin: The "Gatekeeper" Hormone

Insulin acts like a key that unlocks the body's cells so sugar (in the form of glucose) can move into them to be used as energy. Every time you down a carb-laden dessert that makes your blood sugar skyrocket, your pancreas responds by releasing insulin to handle the onslaught of sugar. If you overdo the pasta, breads, or sweets, insulin can deliver only so much of that sugar to your cells, and the excess calories are stored as fat. Worse, constant high levels of blood sugar can lead to what's known as *insulin resistance*, a condition in which cells become less responsive to the hormone. And that's the precursor to diabetes, one of the most effective age accelerators known to man.

BALANCE IT OUT: Just by following the dietary guidelines in this book you'll help your gatekeeper hormone do its job without becoming overwhelmed. By cutting out added sugars and replacing a lot of processed carbohydrates with ancient grains and fresh vegetables, you will avoid the dangerous blood sugar spikes that lead to insulin resistance. Here's an easy step to take immediately: Replace sugary soft drinks with water, lemon water, and unsweetened iced tea. According to a study in the journal *Circulation*, soft drinks account for a full third of the added sugars in our diets, so nixing them is a great start.

Estrogen and Progesterone: The "Cycle Hormones"

These powerful hormones that drive ovulation and menstruation impact many aspects of your life, including your mood, hunger, cravings, libido, and weight. The key to managing those changes and the dreaded PMS symptoms is helping your body reduce estrogen dominance throughout your cycle.

BALANCE IT OUT: Incorporate a regular rotation of specific power foods into your diet to help break down estrogen and usher it from your body. In her book *WomanCode*, Vitti details a comprehensive plan to improve hormonal health, which includes a 4-week jump-start nutrition plan that increases valuable micronutrients at key points in your cycle so your endocrine system produces optimal hormone levels. Give it a try, starting the day after your period ends; if you don't get your period, start Week 1 on a Sunday.

Week 1

Estrogen is increasing. Eat more sprouted and fermented foods to keep estrogen moving. Sauerkraut, kimchi, bean sprouts, and sprouted breads provide your body with key probiotics, particularly indole-3-carbinol, which helps break down estrogen.

Week 2

Estrogen is surging at this point, so use antioxidants to help your liver process it out of your system. Raw juices and fresh vegetables are the ticket. Make a veggie juice from beets, kale, lemon, apple, and ginger, for example. Add more raw fruits and vegetables to your salads and snacks. These foods ensure that your liver gets the crucial micronutrient glutathione, which is required to break down estrogen. "We don't absorb synthetic glutathione well; the only way you can reap the benefits is by eating it," says Vitti.

Week 3

During this transition week, there is a jump in both estrogen and progesterone, and then there's a drop that can affect brain chemistry and mood. To keep your mood stable during this turbulent time, eat more whole grains and greens. They provide B vitamins, the building blocks of serotonin, and soluble fiber, which helps move estrogen out of your body quickly.

Week 4

As hormone levels drop this week, focus on eating more healthy fats (like salmon and avocados) and root vegetables. Both will help stabilize your mood and boost energy. The vitamin A from beets, sweet potatoes, carrots, and pumpkin will help your liver process estrogen.

Ask the Life Stylist

Alisa Vitti, integrative nutritionist, holistic health counselor, hormone expert, founder of FLOliving.com, and author of *WomanCode*

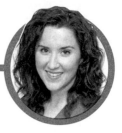

Q > **Is there anything I can do to age-proof my sex drive? I have a strong libido now, but I'm only 35.**

A < You obviously know that your libido can be affected by the changing hormone levels that occur as you get older. But don't worry. There's much you can do to keep desire strong and your sex life healthy. Avoiding weight gain is an important step, and fortunately, many of the strategies to achieve that can also combat hormonal effects on libido. Try eating more healthy fats, like nuts and coconut oil, and protein to help keep your blood sugar steady and mood stable. Strength training (see Chapter 10) can increase testosterone production and your libido. Consider taking an energy-revving B vitamin complex supplement and eating protein-rich foods like eggs and tuna that bring vitamin B to the plate naturally.

Q > **Even though I exercise regularly and follow a strict diet, I can't seem to lose weight. Why isn't normal weight-loss advice working?**

A < Deprivation isn't the answer. Tweak your daily routine with these fixes: Stabilize your blood sugar throughout the day by balancing each meal with a serving of complex carbohydrates, protein, and fat. Split time equally between strength training and cardio, but keep workouts to 30 minutes or less to ensure you don't pump out fat-storing cortisol. And eat a green vegetable (check out the list on pages 82 and 83) at every meal to help your liver detoxify estrogen quickly.

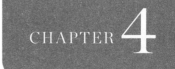

CHAPTER 4

The Meditation Connection/Greater
Awareness Empowers Self-Control

> When I started meditating, I felt more energy . . . I felt healthier and more *comfortable* in my body. The whole world looked better.
> —DAVID LYNCH, FILM DIRECTOR

EVEN THOUGH I HAD BEEN READING STUDIES ABOUT THE benefits of meditation in my job as the editor of a healthy living magazine, I still harbored the notion that meditation was too "woo woo" for a hard-charging type A like me. I was afraid that finding my Zen would dull my edge. But I learned through research and talking to experts that it actually does the opposite: It gives you an edge by reducing stress and making you less reactionary . . . and that means you're less likely to lash out at someone in anger and less likely to react to being upset by thrusting your hand into the cookie jar.

So I got trained in Transcendental Meditation (TM)—twice. Once by a lovely teacher named Betty Jones in Los Angeles, and another time—to reinforce the practice—here in New York through the David Lynch Foundation. (If you aren't familiar with this remarkable organization, please visit davidlynchfoundation.org to learn more. In brief, its mission is to bring science-based stress-reducing techniques like TM to at-risk populations that would otherwise never have the opportunity to learn them: women and girls who are victims of domestic violence, veterans with post-traumatic stress disorder, homeless men, and inner-city kids, among others. Their work is outstanding.)

Practicing TM changed my entire demeanor, so much so that friends started asking if I'd done something different with my hair! I was more level, a little brighter, more in control—and I most definitely did not lose my edge. In fact, my daily practice just made me sharper in the workplace (and every other area of my life). Meditation, after all, teaches you awareness, focus, and control. Those are key skills that lead to the kind of mindful approach to eating that's such an important part of the 20 Pounds Younger program. In the next chapter, you will learn specific techniques for developing mindfulness; in this chapter, we will explore meditation and teach you some simple meditation techniques that will help you master mindfulness. My hope is that, after reading this chapter and trying some "meditation lite" exercises, you'll be intrigued enough to give Transcendental Meditation a try. TM can't be taught by a book, and certainly not through the 20 Pounds Younger program; it requires training with an instructor. But the health benefits, as you'll see, are incredible, and I highly recommend that you explore the practice further on your own. Meanwhile, let's take a look at some common myths about meditation. If you're anything like I was—and I suspect you are—you probably have a few questions and doubts about meditation that I hope to dispel here.

MYTH #1: *Meditation Means Doing Nothing*

If you've ever seen monks in a temple, you may have assumed that they're just sitting there, staring off into space—but that's because you're not a mind reader. "This is a huge misconception," says Adam Burke, PhD, director of The Institute for Holistic Health Studies at San Francisco State University. "Meditation actually does require quite a bit of mental intention and application of awareness. It's definitely not just relaxing." Psychologist Jean Kristeller, PhD, who studies meditation, adds, "It often gets dismissed as just another relaxation technique.

But meditation cultivates mindfulness—you're giving yourself space to observe what's arising in your mind, and to be aware of it, without reacting to it." It's *not* just letting your mind go blank. The mental exercise may come in the form of a mantra (a word or phrase you say over and over) or from paying close attention to your breathing.

MYTH #2: *Meditation Is a Religious Practice*
You *can* make meditation a spiritual experience, but it can also be as nonreligious as a yoga class at your gym. "Meditation does come from cultures where it was affiliated with religious traditions, like Hinduism," says Dr. Burke. "But there are some practices, like mindfulness meditation, that have become very secularized." And if you are a spiritual person—but not a member of the Hindu faith—you can easily adapt your practice to sync with your beliefs (for example, by using one line of a prayer as your mantra), says Life Stylist Gabrielle Bernstein, meditation and Kundalini yoga teacher and *New York Times* bestselling author of *May Cause Miracles* and *Miracles Now.*

MYTH #3: *If My Mind Starts Wandering, I Must Not Be Cut Out for Meditation*
There's a reason it's called a practice: Meditation takes lots of practice! "People will say, 'Oh, I'm not doing it right, because I'm thinking about all of these other things,'" says Dr. Kristeller. "But, no: You *are* doing it right just by becoming aware that you're thinking about other things." So take it as a sign of progress if you notice that your mind wanders, because most of the time, people become so tangled up in their mental mazes that they don't even realize they've lost focus.

MYTH #4: *You Need a Meditation Teacher*
This is true specifically of Transcendental Meditation, which requires in-person training before you can practice, says Bernstein. But you can master other varieties—and there are dozens of them—with the help of a CD, book, or even a smartphone app. On the following pages, you'll find step-by-step instructions for some easy mini meditations to get you started.

MYTH #5: *Meditation Is a Time Suck!*

Transcendental Meditation prescribes a 20-minute practice in the morning and then another 20 minutes in the evening. "Even though that's actually a very short amount of time, it sounds like a lot," acknowledges Dr. Burke. Agree? Then adopt the beginner's motto: Some time is better than none. "Inner peace can be achieved in the time it takes to make a sandwich," says Andy Puddicombe, founder of GetSomeHeadSpace.com. Start off by meditating for 2 or 3 minutes, 5 days a week. Then slowly build up to 10 to 15 minutes. A study from the University of Pennsylvania found that meditating for just 12 minutes a day can improve your mood.

"You don't need to be a Buddhist monk to reap the benefits of mindfulness," says Puddicombe. He says mini meditation breaks throughout the day can clear your mind and help you feel less stress and more control. Commit yourself to giving it a shot tomorrow. Here's how.

In the morning, fine-tune your focus for the day ahead.

Sit in a comfortable chair near a window with your feet flat on the floor and your hands in your lap. Take five slow, deep breaths while gazing straight ahead. Return to a natural breathing rhythm and imagine the sun's rays coming through the window and warming you to your core, its brightness melting away all of your stress and clearing your mind. (If it's a gray day outside, envision a gentle rain washing away your tension.) Enjoy the sensation for a few minutes, then slowly stretch your arms and legs before rising.

During your commute, exercise your senses.

Take a minute to center yourself as you're riding the train or bus (don't try this if you're driving!). Sit up straight and focus on your butt pressing against the seat. Start by listening to the sounds around you—muffled music from someone else's earphones, the buzz of people talking—and then let each of your other senses take center stage for a minute. What do you see, smell, and feel? Now embrace all of your senses simultaneously: Think of them as parts of an orchestra coming together. Notice how everything is always moving and imagine yourself as part of this ever-changing environment, rather than being stressed-out by it.

Reclaim your lunch hour.

Before taking that first bite, spend 2 minutes doing nothing. Just relax and leave work behind. Then make like a *Top Chef* judge and really be aware of what you're eating. Slowly unwrap your meal and take in its aroma. Imagine where the food came from: Envision the ingredients growing on a farm, sprouting from a seed into a vegetable. Chew slowly, and pay attention to how the food feels in your mouth—the taste, texture, and temperature on your tongue. (We'll go into more detail on mindful eating in the next chapter and in Your Mindful Eating Workshop on page 223.)

Drift off to sleep.

Lie in bed with your eyes closed. Take deep breaths as you imagine your mind floating down your body to your feet. Now focus on the pinkie toe of your left foot. Envision an on/off switch for this toe and "power it down" as you would a laptop. Move to the next toe and do the same thing. After each toe has been "shut down," let your mind float back up through your feet and legs to your waist. Repeat the exercise, starting with the small toe of your right foot. Continue powering down as your mind floats up through your legs and waist, but this time, imagine your mind floating all the way up to your head. *Good night. See you in the morning.*

How Meditation Beats Stress

While meditation comes in dozens of forms, they all involve one thing: a heightened state of awareness. That can be a tough concept to grasp, so consider this analogy: At any given time, your thoughts bounce like Ping-Pong balls between the past and the future, stuck on what could have been or fixed on what might be. Rarely do they zero in on what *is*. But research shows that finding your "right now"—as New Age-y as it sounds—can over-haul your body and brain.

Yoga, meditation, tai chi—all of these practices help to elicit what mind-body experts call the "relaxation response." Not to be confused with vegging out, "this is an innate body response that's opposite to the stress response," says Herbert Benson, MD, director emeritus of the Benson-Henry Institute for Mind Body Medicine at Massachusetts General Hospital and a professor of mind-body medicine at Harvard Medical School. "The relaxation response actually changes your genes' expression." When you evoke the relaxation response through meditation, your DNA is translated into active RNA, which kicks off the production of proteins that counteract the harmful effects of mental tension, says Dr. Benson.

Compare that to stress, which activates proteins that exacerbate—or even cause—diseases and disorders responsible for 60 to 90 percent of doctors' visits, he says. This includes anxiety and depression, heart attacks, strokes, irritable bowel syndrome, PMS, and insomnia, among other health issues. "People feel that meditation is an Eastern—or non-Western, nonscientific—approach that's not part of our culture," says Dr. Benson, "when truly we all have the relaxation response within us."

Anything that can conquer stress will also target the health problems associated with it. In fact, University of Hawaii, UCLA, and Maharishi University of Management researchers found that people who meditated experienced a 48 percent decrease in symptoms associated with depression. And in another study, people who reported reduced anxiety as a result of meditation saw a simultaneous drop in their levels of C-reactive protein, a substance linked to inflammation of the arteries.

Two things are necessary to enter this state of body-boosting relaxation: The first is repetition, and it will help you master the second, which is keeping your mind from wandering. "Repetition can be a word, a sound, a prayer, a phrase, or a movement," says Dr. Benson. "One could focus simply on the breath."

In Transcendental Meditation, repetition comes in the form of a secret mantra—usually a Sanskrit word or phrase—that's assigned to you by your instructor. You simply say it over and over, returning back to it whenever a random thought pops into your head. Your mantra isn't supposed to have any personal significance; the goal is simply to equip you with a soothing sound that helps you break the chain of everyday thinking. By contrast, in Kundalini meditation, you use a variety of meaningful phrases, depending on the goal of your meditation session. One example is *sat nam,* which means "truth identified."

You can, of course, choose your own mantra, as long as it uplifts you. "All words carry an energy," says Bernstein.

Before you discount that as a bunch of B.S., try my little experiment: Mentally repeat a word you hate, then do the same with a gentler word, like "love." Feel the difference?

THREE MANTRAS THAT INSPIRE

Take these uplifting examples for a spin.

If You Seek a Sense of Calm

Love (on the inhale), *peace* (on the exhale)

If You Want to Forgive Someone

I forgive you (on the inhale), *I release you* (on the exhale)

If You Want to Connect with Yourself

Soham ("soooo" on the inhale, "hammmm" on the exhale, meaning "I am that" in Sanskrit)

If you'd rather sit in silence, you can just zero in on your breathing or even the pattern of your pulse. "Breathe in four beats through your nose and one beat out through your nose," suggests Bernstein. "That can connect you right to your breath." (She says this exercise is especially good for newcomers.) Another option: Simply inhale for 5 seconds, then exhale for 5 seconds. Or, if you want to incorporate your pulse into your practice, place your index finger on your wrist, over your pulse point, and your thumb underneath. "Just breathe long and deep, and check into your pulse," says Bernstein. "That can be very powerful."

The point of all this repetition—whether you're using a mantra or just observing your body's natural rhythms—is to keep yourself tuned in to the present moment and not lost in your thoughts. "If your thoughts are chaotic—you start to think about your to-do list—you can go right back into that mantra," says Bernstein. That's much different than trying to shove your grocery list out of your mind. You're simply replacing your thoughts, rather than fighting them. (This is a strategy you'll learn to apply to food cravings in The Mindful Eating Workshop, page 223.)

As unnatural as this may seem, redirecting your thoughts is a lot less mentally taxing than actively pushing them away. "The practice itself is relatively easy," says Stephan Bodian, author of *Meditation for Dummies*, who compares meditation to running. Just as you have to train your body before you can run a marathon, you have to train your mind to be attentive and aware.

TRAINING YOUR MIND FOR AWARENESS

What's the point of elevating your awareness? The idea is to break through your superficial thoughts, which are the ones that often dominate your day. "The mind has layers, with the 'chattering mind' at the top, more stable patterns of emotions and thoughts below that, and 'inner wisdom' below that," says Dr. Kristeller. Think about your mind like a river: "Thoughts in the chattering mind tend to come and go very quickly, like the ripples in a rapidly moving stream of water," she says. "A feeling or thought may be more enduring, like watching a branch or leaf floating on a slowly running river."

Meditation helps you simply observe those leaves passing by, without reacting to them, analyzing them, or even trying to pluck them out of the water before shifting your focus to another leaf. "As you watch the river of thoughts, you note, 'twig, twig,' following the twig until it drifts out of sight, perhaps fully experiencing it, but not analyzing it," says Dr. Kristeller. It's okay if a judgment or two slips in, as long as you acknowledge it without elaborating on it. Compare that to most people's normal style of associative thinking: *Oh, what a pretty leaf. That reminds me—I have to water my plants tomorrow. Oh, wow, that's a candy wrapper floating by. Why do people throw trash in the river? Oh darn, I forgot to put out the trash. . . .*

After you tune in to all the mental clatter and then quiet it with a mantra or by focusing on your breath, you can more clearly observe your thoughts and emotions—the things that often drive you to eat or make the choices you do. By sitting with these emotions, rather than reacting to them, you start to connect with your own innate inner wisdom, the part of you that knows what your body needs—including at mealtimes, says Dr. Kristeller.

Eventually, these mental practices will become second nature—and you may even find yourself applying them off the cushion. "I meditate throughout the day, all the time," says Bernstein. "For instance, if I'm feeling really stressed-out, I'll just do a really quick meditation at my desk: four breaths in, breathe out for one. I'll do that for 1 minute."

Perhaps the most important place to apply your meditative skills is at the dinner table. As part of Dr. Kristeller's Mindfulness-Based Eating Awareness Training (MB-EAT) program, a version of which you'll find on page 223, she has people practice "mini meditations" before—or even in the middle of—meals and snacks. "It's just a few minutes of breath awareness to calm yourself," she explains, "and to say, 'What's going on here? Why am I reaching for the box of cookies? Do I really want them?'" If you're midway through a meal, you might focus on your breathing while checking in with your body: Are you full? Are you hungry? Do you want to stop eating your mashed potatoes so you can save room for dessert? Are you still even tasting the mashed potatoes? (For complete instructions on mini meditations, see page 229.)

ASK THE LIFE STYLIST

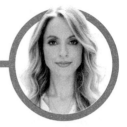

Gabrielle Bernstein, meditation and Kundalini yoga teacher and *New York Times* bestselling author of *May Cause Miracles* and *Miracles Now*

Q > Can I meditate at the office without looking crazy?

A < This is one of my favorite places to meditate! If I'm super stressed, with a ton of things on my plate, I'll do a really quick meditation at my desk: I breathe in four strokes (beats), then out one, continuing to alternate for a full 60 seconds. The effect: I feel instantly energized and refocused. Meditation is a great tool for pivoting out of a negative frame of mind and into a more peaceful one—fast. And no one even has to know you're doing it.

Q > Meditation seems boring. Aren't you just doing the same thing every day?

A < It's smart to sit in the same spot every time you meditate, but that doesn't mean all sessions have to be identical. I recommend setting a unique intention for each practice; think of this as your goal for however long you decide to commit to relaxing. Your intention could be something as simple as releasing stress, calming down, or even allowing yourself to forgive someone. But don't feel obligated to decide on a goal: It can be equally profound to leave your session open to creative ideas and possibilities, since meditation is one of the greatest ways to allow your creative intuition to come forward.

THE *MEDICATION* IN MEDITATION

Transcendental Meditation—the kind that I've been trained in—is the most widely studied method. (In his book *Transcendence,* Norman E. Rosenthal, MD, who is a clinical professor of psychiatry at Georgetown Medical School, says he's counted 340 peer-reviewed articles on TM.) That means the benefits aren't just tough-to-put-your-finger-on things, like inner peace or a sense of Zen. People who are unfamiliar with meditation often assume it's as hokey as "as seen on TV" products, but the truth is, TM is probably more scientifically supported than some of the medical treatments that most of us accept.

Blood pressure control is perhaps the most lauded perk of getting into the meditation zone. "Transcendental Meditation is very, very focused on stress reduction and lowering blood pressure," says Bernstein. In a Medical College of Georgia study, researchers asked teenagers with "high normal" blood pressure—that is, close to the upper limit of what's considered healthy—to practice TM for 15 minutes, twice a day, for 2 months, while a similar group of adolescents attended a series of 1-hour talks about diet and exercise. At the end of the study, the kids who didn't meditate showed a slight *increase* in blood pressure, while the meditative teens' blood pressure levels had dropped. Similarly, when the teenagers played a high-intensity car racing video game, those who'd been regularly meditating experienced a smaller spike in heart rate.

A racing heart is one of the classic sign of stress—it's a side effect of your sympathetic nervous system kicking into gear. When you encounter a stressor, even something as incidental as a loud noise, your heart naturally starts pumping harder. The big question: How fast do you recover? "Meditators get a brisk uptick in blood pressure, but it comes back down very quickly," says Dr. Rosenthal. Compare that with nonmeditators, whose blood pressure shoots up in response to a stressor, stays elevated longer, and then randomly spikes a few more times, even after the alarming incident has passed. By practicing meditation, "you're shifting your stress response system to a more stable position, so it doesn't get activated by triggers," explains Dr. Rosenthal.

That study group was a relatively healthy bunch: young, with blood pressure in the recommended range. So how would TM impact a higher risk group? The short answer: Transcendental Meditation can help undo the health-threatening effects of heart disease. That's a pretty big promise—and it's totally supported by science. "In the early phases of cardiovascular disease, the lining of the arteries is beginning to thicken, often because of chronic high blood pressure," says Dr. Rosenthal. "Imagine a river where the water is becoming more turbulent. That would damage the riverbank." But this arterial hardening doesn't have to be permanent—and TM is one way to hit the reverse button.

In a study published in the journal *Stroke*, scientists recruited 138 African Americans—a population known to have an elevated risk of heart disease—who'd been diagnosed with high blood pressure. They were randomly assigned to one of two groups: Half practiced Transcendental Meditation for 20 minutes twice a day, while the others took a course in health education and spent the same amount of time doing leisure activities (such as reading or exercising) each day. After several months, the meditation group showed a significant decrease in the thickness of the lining of their carotid arteries, suggesting that the damage inflicted by high blood pressure was beginning to reverse itself. How'd the other folks fare? The lining of their carotid arteries *thickened*—which means their arterial trouble had only continued progressing.

The carotid artery is what shuttles blood to your brain—another area of your body that receives big-time benefits from Transcendental Meditation. At any given moment, your brain is relaying multiple signals, and those signals aren't always in sync or consistent. Interestingly, TM has been shown to remedy this by increasing "brain wave coherence," which means that different areas of the brain emit the same wavelengths at the same time. "That's associated with more competency," says Dr. Rosenthal. "Successful business people and more competent athletes have been shown to have more brain coherence."

MEDITATE—WITH YOUR FEET

You don't have to sit on a cushion to get your meditation fix; you can do it while walking. "Mindful walking has a long history within meditative traditions, including both Buddhist and Christian," says psychologist Jean Kristeller, PhD. It's an easy way to practice being mindful while also burning calories, and it can help you learn to focus on your breath while exercising. It can be done at any pace. Here, Dr. Kristeller takes you through it step by step.

1. **Stand with your feet shoulder-width apart.** Close your eyes, or rest your gaze on a spot on the ground 3 to 4 feet in front of you. Notice how your feet feel on the ground (remove your shoes if you wish). Soften your knees so blood can flow easily into and out of your legs.

2. **Notice your breath, feeling the air moving into the center of your body.** Make sure your abdomen is expanding before your chest does as you inhale, then releasing gently as you exhale.

3. **Now return your attention to your feet.** Imagine you have four points of contact with the ground: the inside and outside of the front half of your feet and the inside and outside of the back half. Slowly rock back and forth until you feel your weight distributed equally over all four points of your feet.

4. **Start walking at your normal pace.** After a few minutes, slow down as much as possible: Gently move your weight onto your left foot, slowly lifting your right foot and placing it in front of you. Then gently shift your weight onto your right foot as you slowly lift your left foot and place it in front of you. Notice how your balance changes from moment to moment. Just relax and move, being attentive to each movement of shifting, lifting, swinging, placing.

5. **Now try this at a faster pace, somewhere between the very slow speed and your normal speed.** For 5 minutes, alternate between your very slow speed, moderate speed, and normal speed.

6. **Finally, stand still and silent for several moments as your heart rate comes down.** What does it feel like to stop the momentum of movement? What is it like to be still? Return your focus to your four points of contact with the ground, noticing your breath in the center of your body.

This neural synchrony continues even after you stop meditating—an effect seen in novice and seasoned practitioners alike. The result? You're more in control of your emotions and less impulsive, which, as you can imagine, is an obvious perk for people who struggle with stress eating. "Trying to lose weight on your own is a major challenge," says Dr. Rosenthal. "You have to be very disciplined, coordinated, and competent—plan your meals, do your food shopping, make sure there are healthy choices in your fridge. The more brain coherence you have—and the more competent you are—the better off you're going to be, in terms of your diet."

10 TIPS: MAKE THE MOST OUT OF MEDITATION

Every person's practice is different. You may find that you prefer a certain style of meditation or that you favor a specific time of day for doing it. That's perfectly acceptable—encouraged, even. You *want* to figure out the ideal practice for you, as you're more likely to stick with a method of meditation that you love. That said, it's easy for beginners to feel lost, with no clue where to start or even how to sit. Here's how to set yourself up for success.

SUCCESS STRATEGY #1: *Pick a Time of Day and Stick with It*

You can meditate whenever you want, as long as you're consistent. However, experts say that if you're only going to take time out once a day, the morning is ideal. Why? Most of us tend to be more routine-oriented in the a.m. compared to the evening, making it fairly easy to add a few minutes of meditation to the mix. "You won't go to work without brushing your teeth or taking a shower," says Bernstein. "But you could maybe go to bed without doing those things." Think of morning meditation as a mental shower to clear your day. "Meditating in the morning can help clear your mind so that you can do things faster and with more focus," says Frank Lipman, MD, an integrative medicine specialist. "You can actually end up with more time."

SUCCESS STRATEGY #2: *Commit to 40 Days of Practice*

During your first couple of attempts at meditating, you may find your mind racing, zigzagging around like a rat in a maze. That's discouraging—but don't give up. "Consistency is crucial," says Bernstein. "Choose a method, and then commit to 40 days of practice. In that 40-day period, you'll create new neural pathways in your brain, so you really start to see the longer-lasting change." Chances are, you won't want to quit once you truly give your body a chance to adapt.

SUCCESS STRATEGY #3: *Stake Out a Meditation Space*

Your brain craves routine. You probably sleep, eat, and work in the same places, day in and day out, so your brain starts to anticipate—and prepare for—those behaviors. So if you make your practice predictable—for example, by always sitting on the same cushion, in the same corner of your sunroom—your mind may more readily enter a state of relaxation, says Dr. Burke. One guideline: Make sure your meditation zone is a quiet space.

SUCCESS STRATEGY #4: *Watch Your Posture*

Serious practitioners often sit on a simple cushion. But if you find it difficult to maintain good posture without lower-back support, you're better off in a chair or even on a couch, says Dr. Burke. "Comfortable seating is the main thing," he says. (You can even meditate in your bed, if that's where you're comfortable, notes Bernstein.) If you opt for the floor, try sitting cross-legged while keeping your back straight; this posture is called "easy pose" in Kundalini meditation, and it makes it easier to breathe properly.

SUCCESS STRATEGY #5: *Don't Panic If Thoughts Pop Up*

Catch yourself recapping a recent episode of *Orange Is the New Black?* Stressing over a deadline at work? You could freak out and decide you're not cut out for meditation, but that'd just be feeding the very cycle of thinking that you're trying to overcome. Simply acknowledge the thought without judgment, and refocus on your mantra or your breathing. It's really as simple as that.

SUCCESS STRATEGY #6: *Set a Timer*

Just as random thoughts can invade your practice, it's easy to start obsessing over how many minutes you've been meditating. By setting a timer, you thwart some of the "I wonder what time it is" thinking, says Dr. Kristeller. (And that translates to less mental clutter threatening your relaxation.) She suggests placing it in a nearby room; that way, you can hear it but it doesn't startle you when it sounds. If your spouse or children are home, make sure to point out the timer to discourage them from disturbing you.

SUCCESS STRATEGY #7: *Breathe Properly*

Even if you're focusing on a mantra—not the cycle of your inhales and exhales—you need to breathe properly in order to elicit the relaxation response. You'll know you're breathing through your diaphragm (as you should be) if your shoulders don't move up and down and your stomach and ribs expand, says Dr. Kristeller. At first, you may need to consciously take deep breaths to get in the zone, but your breathing will quickly fall into its own natural rhythm.

SUCCESS STRATEGY #8: *Don't Meditate on a Full Stomach*

Of course, any meditation is better than no meditation. But if possible, avoid carving out your meditation time right after a big meal, says Dr. Kristeller. Why? You'll just be uncomfortable, making it hard to tune out your inner experience and slip into a state of relaxation. Similarly, you should avoid meditating near bedtime, when you're getting sleepy, since you could drift off during your practice.

SUCCESS STRATEGY #9: *Set Aside Any Expectations*

Every day is different, which means that every time you practice, you'll be in a very different state of mind. Read: You can't expect an awesome session every day—and if you do, you'll only set yourself up for self-criticism, which is exactly the opposite of what you want to gain from meditation. Of course, it's okay to set an intention for your practice, such as stress relief or forgiveness, but that doesn't mean holding yourself to the same standard every day.

SUCCESS STRATEGY #10: *Ease Out of Meditation Gradually*

You don't slip into a state of relaxation within seconds, so you shouldn't rush out of it, either. Abruptly opening your eyes can be jarring—the opposite of how you should feel after 20 minutes of meditating. So open your eyes slowly, gradually shift your focus back to the room, and then transition to the next part of your day.

THREE TAKEAWAYS TO TRY TODAY

1. **Don't get discouraged.** Meditation takes practice. If you notice that your mind is wandering, that's proof of your progress in developing awareness.

2. **Pick an uplifting mantra.** Can't think of one? Try "peace" or *soham* ("so" on the inhale, "hammm" on exhale).

3. **Start off with a quick at-the-office meditation,** a walking meditation, or several mini meditations during the day.

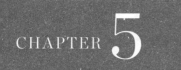
Eat, Drink, and Be Mindful/

In a World Filled with Sugary Temptation, This Is the Secret to Weight Control

Our *three basic needs,* for food and security and love, are so mixed and mingled and entwined that we cannot straightly think about one without the others.

–FOOD WRITER M. F. K. FISHER

"MINDFULNESS" HAS BECOME SOMETHING OF A BUZZWORD over the past few years. Most of us associate it with yoga mats and mantras, but do you really know what it means to be mindful?

Actually, you practice mindfulness every day; you just may not realize you're doing it. You're being mindful when you buckle your seat belt or say no to the third glass of wine because you have to drive home. You're being mindful when you choose the hot tea over that yummy sweet mocha toffee latte that contains 420 mostly empty calories. You're engaging powerful mindfulness muscles when you rewrite that vitriol-laced e-mail to a coworker before hitting send. See, mindfulness isn't so foreign after all. But applied more, well, *mindfully,* it can be a really effective tool for weight loss.

A lot of experts define mindfulness as bringing awareness and attention to any experience without getting tangled up in judgment. "Why would this make a difference?" asks psychologist Jean Kristeller, PhD. "Because our reactivity—our sense of being out of control about things—comes from judgment: "This is something I want more of. This is something I want to avoid." This happens extremely quickly, and once it happens, we feel like we don't have any choice, any alternative way of relating to something." But the more mindful you are, the less susceptible you may be to the temptation of immediate rewards, suggests a 2013 study in the journal *Emotion*.

As I mentioned earlier, one of the most functional—and life-changing—applications of mindfulness happens at the table, where you're inundated with a million different signals to shovel it in. There are the external cues to eat—things like the sight or smell of food, or friends chowing down—which are compounded by internal prompts to dig in, such as a negative emotion or even just the perception that those mashed potatoes look OMG-amazing. "Mindfulness encourages you to be aware of both types of cues while you're eating," says Katie Rickel, PhD, a clinical psychologist and weight-loss expert who works at a weight-management facility in Durham, North Carolina. "You're not trying to change or evaluate them. You're just noticing them—and not letting them interfere with your decisions about eating."

Let's start with an example of how most of us normally eat. You spot a tray of macadamia nut cookies and almost automatically make a judgment: "Those cookies look amazing, but it'd be wrong of me to eat them." If you accept that judgment as the final word—an indisputable fact—you now have two options: You can continue to stare longingly at the cookies without touching them, or you can eat one and feel horribly guilty. Neither of those sounds too fun, right? Keep in mind: Judgment isn't always negative. When you spot those same cookies, your autopilot mind might conclude, "Wow, I love cookies! Dig in, sister!" You might start eating the cookies without paying attention to their taste because you just generally like macadamia nut cookies, so your autopilot tells you to start devouring them. These scenarios are what we call *mindless* eating.

In both situations, you took your initial reaction as fact: "Cookies are bad." Or, "cookies are so incredible I must eat them." But what if neither of those thoughts is true? What if you paused for a moment to consider whether there are, in fact, alternative ways to think about those cookies?

Imagine that you zero in on that same tray of cookies, but instead of reflexively grabbing a few, you acknowledge that initial judgment—*I want those cookies, ASAP*—but decide that you won't immediately accept the "cookies are good, therefore I eat" conclusion as absolute truth. You still approach the table, but before you take a couple, you check them out. That's when you realize they're not homemade. In fact, they're the hard, store-bought cookies you aren't particularly fond of. Still, you decide to sample one—and yep, just as you suspected, it's totally dry and tasteless. You put it down.

That's what you call *mindful* eating. It's not about resistance. It's not about deprivation. It's about deciding: Do I really want this? What is my body—not my mind—telling me? And if the answer is, "Yes, I do, in fact, want this cookie," then you eat the cookie. And you enjoy it.

Sound easy? You know it's not. Deciding whether or not to eat a cookie is not the same as deciding whether or not to buckle your seat belt. But with practice and some tricks of the mindfulness trade, you can learn to do it really, really effectively. If you're game to start right now, jump to the appendix on page 223; that's where you'll find Your Mindful Eating Workshop, specially created for this book by Dr. Kristeller. It's a life-altering 6-week program that will guide you, step-by-step, to mastering more mindful eating. Or you can continue reading here and start the workshop tonight as part of your 20 Pounds Younger homework assignment.

Tuning In to Your Body

Is that a headache coming on? I could really go for a latte right now. I wonder if I'm addicted to caffeine? I do notice it helps me push harder in the gym. And speaking of, I really hope Julie is at spin class tonight . . . .

Sound familiar? As women, we tend to be pretty in tune with ourselves. We usually know how our bodies feel at any given moment and why and how we can make things better (or at least we think we do). Yet in one area, many of us are astonishingly out of touch: recognizing when we're hungry and when we're full. "Some experts think that one of the reasons people become obese, or start to have problems with food, is that there is something broken," says Dr. Kristeller. "The theory is that their hunger signals just don't happen, or don't happen in a way that's particularly easy to tune in to."

And while you may not have reached the point of total impairment, your signals may be a little staticky. If you've ever thought, "Hmm, I *guess* I'm hungry, so I *guess* I'll eat," or, "Well, it's lunchtime, so I'd better buy a sandwich," then this may very well be you. Compare this to the I-know-what-I-need confident statements you make when eating based on internal cues:

"I always stop eating when I start feeling full."

"I push back the plate when I want to leave room for dessert."

"If food doesn't taste good anymore, I just don't eat it."

Part of the problem is that lots of physical sensations and emotions can masquerade as hunger. "If people are thirsty, they often think they're hungry. If they're tired, they often think they're hungry," says Dr. Rickel. "When people are anxious, they often think they're hungry." (Think back to the connection between cortisol and appetite, discussed in Chapter 3.) She adds: "It's very, very difficult to use hunger and fullness to make decisions about what and how much we eat. Our cues for eating are so warped by the time we reach adulthood. Hunger is a funny word, because it so rarely refers to physical hunger." Think about it: Even our expressions for feeling nervous—"I have a lump in my throat" and "I've got butterflies in my stomach"—are related to our gastrointestinal system.

Why does it matter whether your body or the amount of food on your plate tells you to eat? Because it may play a critical role in the size of your jeans. People with a body mass index of 25 or higher—the point at which

HOW MINDFULNESS RETRAINS YOUR BRAIN

After 6 weeks of mindfulness training, participants in a study reported experiencing the following noteworthy changes, according to an article published in the journal *Complementary Therapies in Medicine*.

16 percent decrease in the tendency to eat out of control

39 percent decrease in hunger

43 percent decrease in binge eating incidences

26 percent decrease in depression

35 percent decrease in anxiety

Source: *Complementary Therapies in Medicine*

they're considered overweight—rely on external stop-and-go signals (for example, whether there is food visible or the plate is empty, rather than listening to their own internal cues) much more than normal-weight eaters do, according to a study in the journal *Obesity*.

Learning to discern what your body is saying to you—whether that message is "feed me now, dammit!" or "set the fork down!"—is what Dr. Kristeller calls "inner wisdom." Not only are you recognizing the inherent value of your body's signals, but you're also making the important distinction between emotional states, like anxiety or anger, and actual hunger—all without berating yourself for feeling a need to feed when you're in a real funk.

What Does Judgment Have to Do with Food?

Perhaps you think about judgment only in the context of a divine power. Or maybe the word calls to mind a certain bitchy girlfriend. But as the adage goes, you really are your own worst critic—especially when it comes to your body or what you put on your plate. As women, we are constantly—and often subconsciously—evaluating everything we do or encounter, says Jennifer Daubenmier, PhD, an assistant professor at the Osher Center for Integrative Medicine at the University of California–San Francisco. "We experience things through the filter of our likes and dislikes, wanting certain things, wishing things could be different."

For example:

OMG, I have to order those cheesy fries. They look ah-mazing!

Wow, my butt looks fat in these jeans. I knew I shouldn't have eaten that pasta last night.

I've been so bad already today, I may as well just eat this fried chicken for dinner.

Why, why, why did I eat that doughnut? Ugh, I'm disgusted with myself. I just wish I could get skinny.

I am craving sugar so much that I could eat an entire bag of chocolate. I think I will.

I hate green beans. I'll just have the loaded baked potato instead.

Just as you need to toss out your black-and-white, good-and-bad view of food, you also need to realize that a thought is only that: a thought. It doesn't have to exert power over you. "Mindfulness is about being present to all of these thoughts and judgments," says Dr. Daubenmier. "And when we become aware of those judgments, we can see them as just passing thoughts, instead of glomming onto them."

In the traditional dieting world, weight-loss programs teach you to handle these thoughts through distraction—say, by knitting or reading a book when you want to inhale a bag of chips—or by trying to change your thoughts. "The idea behind this approach is that your thoughts might not be accurate," says Heather Niemeier, PhD, an associate professor of psychology at the University of Wisconsin-Whitewater. Often called control-based strategies, you might be told to banish junk food from your refrigerator; follow a very structured, consistent eating plan; reframe your cravings as figments of your imagination; or, if that fails, just distract yourself from them.

This is the approach that most of us know—and, unfortunately, it doesn't seem to work all that well. (That's why you won't find it in *20 Pounds Younger*.) Sure, the standard control-based strategies may effectively lessen the discomfort of cravings, but they don't give you one important tool: a sense of control over your urges to eat. In other words, this run-of-the-mill approach doesn't really deal with the thoughts that drive you to eat; it just tells you to shove those thoughts out of your mind. Anybody who's ever experienced a craving knows that's one tall order—in fact, trying to cast off your cravings may just crank up their mental volume. And if your attempts to distract yourself don't work, you may end up feeling like a failure, then throw your hands in the air and overeat.

In the past few years, researchers have begun exploring an alternative way of dealing with intrusive thoughts about food: acceptance. It sounds simple enough, but it's actually a three-pronged approach.

1. You recognize that it's hard to control your thoughts and feelings.
2. You increase your awareness—and acceptance—of these internal experiences.
3. You take a mental step back from your thoughts, so they don't wield so much power over your actions.

"You could have the thought 'I feel fat,' and instead of trying to change that thought, you learn to accept it and gain distance from it," explains Dr. Niemeier. You learn to experience your cravings without acting on them.

This approach is all about validating, rather than altering, your thoughts: If you feel fat today, that's a real experience that can hold sway over your day, whether or not you're actually overweight. Or if you're craving a giant chocolate bar, your body may not physically need it, but your mind really thinks it does. "It's not really about shoving thoughts aside," says Dr. Rickel. "It's just about noticing them and being curious about your thoughts, rather than immediately taking them for truth." Once you accept that your internal world is real—and stop constantly trying to change it—you'll free yourself from a lot of the stress of dieting. And by realizing that your thoughts and impulses don't define you or always require a physical response, you'll renew your sense of control over your body and actions. That's critical to weight-loss success.

As odd as this strategy may sound, you probably already practice acceptance all the time—just outside the context of eating. "We have thoughts on a daily basis, constantly, that we don't follow through on," says Dr. Niemeier. For example, every person on the planet has been in a boring meeting and thought, *I want to run out of here.* But do you do it? No. So why do you have to obey the urge to hit the drive-thru or finish off a bag of candy? Some thoughts are more powerful than others (chocolate cravings come to mind), but that doesn't mean you're powerless over them.

In a Drexel University study, people were given transparent boxes of Hershey's Kisses, which they were instructed to keep with them for 48 hours without eating the chocolate. Some participants were told to tackle cravings by distracting themselves or shifting their thinking; others were instructed to simply notice their urge to eat, accept it, and then mentally distance themselves from the impulse. The outcome: The people who practiced acceptance were better able to cope with their cravings, especially if food tended to hold a lot of sway over their behavior and feelings. This was only a 2-day trial, but the researchers speculate that acceptance-based strategies would be even more effective in the real world, outside of a laboratory setting.

You're not trying to cover up your cravings, which you can do only for so long. Instead, "you're going to ride out the wave," says Dr. Niemeier. "You need to sit with the craving and realize that it will not overwhelm you." As counterintuitive as it sounds, you're not going to do that by playing a computer game or going for a walk.

You really have to let your mind and body feel the urge to eat while you distance yourself from the emotional part of it. "Take an observer's perspective on the craving," says Dr. Niemeier. Evaluate it as objectively as you would the weather: What does it look like? Does your craving have a color? What's happening inside your body? She compares the exercise to coddling a crying baby: "You can't try to get rid of it. You just hold it compassionately," she says. "Experience it decreasing, rather than trying to avoid it. Most people notice a lessening of the craving within 10 or 20 minutes." This makes sense: We're most susceptible to our brain's demands during the first 20 minutes after a stressful event—the amount of time it takes for mood-regulating serotonin to bounce back and stress hormones to start to fall away.

One way to distance yourself from irritating urges is to take a step back and ask yourself, "What's my emotional state right now, and why?" (For example: "I'm feeling humiliated because my boss embarrassed me during a staff meeting.") "It becomes more of an inquiry into what triggered the overeating," says Dr. Daubenmier. "It can become a learning opportunity—and a way to extend compassion toward oneself."

Instead of beating yourself up for that potato chip mishap if you do care, treat yourself the way you would a child who's had a bad day at school: Figure out exactly what the upsetting incident was, and ask yourself exactly how it made you feel. If you can understand *why* you want to mainline a pint of mint chocolate chip ice cream, you can figure out what your body really needs. Maybe you'll realize you're super stressed and decide that yoga is a better fix than ice cream. Or perhaps you'll conclude that you really do need a snack, but a piece of fresh fruit would suffice.

3 WAYS TO BEAT MINDLESS MUNCHING

Banish hunger. "Skipping meals sets you up for intense cravings," says Susan Kraus, RD, a nutritionist at Hackensack University Medical Center in New Jersey. Unless you're the rare woman who is completely in tune with her hunger, you need to establish an eating schedule. "This is where preplanning comes in," says Katie Rickel, PhD, a clinical psychologist and weight-loss expert who works at a weight-management facility in Durham, North Carolina. "You're not left in the moment to judge how much to eat." Plus, skipping meals can lead to dangerous thoughts like, "I didn't have breakfast, so I can have this giant piece of cake." It's better to eat a consistent number of calories by the clock than to eat with abandon whenever the mood strikes.

Identify triggers. Keep a detailed food log, recording your moods, what stresses you out, and how hungry you feel before eating. Once you've identified the things that drive you to raid your candy stash, you can react productively instead of eating sweets.

Drink something. The hypothalamus, your brain's control center for mood- and food-related signals, detects thirst as well as hunger. So gulp a glass of water or hot tea (make it decaf—caffeine can trigger the release of stress hormones) and see if the craving passes.

The benefits of accepting your thoughts are immediate—you gain control over your present craving or stop emotional eating in its tracks—as well as long lasting: Over time, you may find that as you learn to accept your cravings, they start cropping up less frequently. In a 2010 study in the journal *Appetite*, dieters who mastered mindfulness and acceptance strategies reported significantly fewer cravings over a 7-week period than those who only focused on healthy eating and exercise. Acceptance also reduced the study participants' loss of control when bombarded with cues to eat.

Success Secrets for Mindful Eating

Mindful eating may not be a mainstream weight-loss tactic (yet), but that doesn't mean it's unsupported by science. In a 2013 Kent State University study, researchers found that mindfulness strategies—for example, paying close attention to the taste and smell of food, and attending to hunger and fullness—significantly increased people's satiety after a meal. Another study showed that dieters who still practiced mindfulness techniques after completing a weight-loss program continued dropping weight. So how can you bring these skills to the table? Start with these secrets to success; then, when you're ready, try the 6-week mindfulness workshop program found in the appendix (see page 223).

ELIMINATE DISTRACTIONS

We live in a world where the ability to multitask is considered resume-worthy. But eating while working, answering e-mails, or doing other tasks can make you consume more than you need. A study in the *American Journal of Clinical Nutrition* found that people who played solitaire during lunch felt less full than undistracted eaters and ate significantly more when offered cookies just half an hour later. So make your meal strictly about eating: Banish the TV, iPad, smartphone, or book from the table, period.

PAY ATTENTION TO PORTIONS

People who eat mindlessly often prefer to remain in a state of ignorance, with no knowledge of serving sizes or the number of calories in foods. But in order to give your body what it needs, you need to face the facts. "How many M&M's is a portion? How many chips?" says Lesley Lutes, PhD, an associate professor of psychology at East Carolina University. "Take it out, put it on your plate." In her experience, people are often surprised—in a good way. "They thought a portion was just 3 or 4 chips," she says. "They felt so guilty about what they were eating that they'd just stick their hand in the bag and keep eating. But we want you to celebrate food." The first step? Understanding—and consciously choosing—what you eat.

PUT YOUR FOOD ON DISPLAY

When you eat straight out of the bag, what happens? (1) You don't stop eating until the bag is empty, and (2) you have no idea how much food you actually shoveled in. "People consume a lot more calories if they're not focused on the food," says Dr. Lutes. "Seeing the food—and seeing the portion size—actually helps you feel more full." So regardless of how much or how little you're eating, use a plate or a bowl. That way, your mind will register that you're eating—and you'll expand the sensory experience (and pleasure) of your meal. "We eat first with our eyes," says Dr. Rickel. "We have to gain some pleasure from the visual appearance of food—otherwise, watching Food Network shows would be totally boring." (This is also why we like to post our meals on Instagram.) Another trick that helps some people: Leave a bit of food on your plate. By conditioning yourself to stop eating before the empty plate signals that you're "full," you'll gain the confidence that you can overcome visual cues to keep eating.

APPRECIATE YOUR FOOD

I know it seems hokey, but before or during your meal, take a moment to think about where your food came from—for example, "This piece of fruit started as a seed, which was planted by a farmer or blown by the wind. Sunlight gave that seed the energy to grow, then someone tended the plant as it matured, harvested the fruit, and delivered it to me." "This makes the experience more whole, rather than just stuffing food into your mouth without thinking about it," says Dr. Rickel. Plus, it's much easier to trace the path of "real" food than it is the heavily processed stuff, which may actually be a little gross to think about in too much detail. "This could probably help you choose cleaner, more whole foods," she says.

START OFF EATING SLOWLY

You probably think eating mindfully means eating at a snail's pace. But that's only true in the beginning. "For teaching purposes, we slow it down," says Dr. Daubenmier. "But with practice, you don't necessarily have to eat in slow motion." As Dr. Rickel points out, "If you took every single bite of every single meal mindfully, then you wouldn't get anything else done during the day." So sure, when you're learning to be mindful, it's helpful to slow down your shoveling. But eventually, tuning in to the experience of eating will become so second nature that you won't have to dine at a grandma pace. One easy way to help you keep a reasonable pace: Put your utensils down and your hands in your lap between bites.

PRETEND YOU'RE A FOOD CRITIC

Your job isn't just to hoover down the food on your plate—you have to take note of the presentation, the nuances of every flavor, and how satisfying each item is. "When you bite into a grape, all of these juices come out—and there are sensations you'd totally miss if you just stuffed a handful of grapes into your mouth," says Dr. Rickel. "Try to follow the first bite down your esophagus and into your belly, and take a moment to notice whether you feel one grape more energetic." In mindful eating workshops, people first practice this with just three or four raisins (see Your Mindful Eating Workshop on page 223). "That really brings people's attention down to their sensory experience," says Dr. Daubenmier. "They really notice the texture, the smell, and the thoughts that come up."

OBSERVE YOUR INNER EXPERIENCE

You can drag out your meal for 2 hours, but all of that extra time doesn't mean a thing if you aren't paying attention to what's happening inside your body and mind. To truly be mindful, you need to take note of every sensation and urge: *How do I know when I'm hungry? What sensations do I experience? What does it feel like when I'm emotionally, but not physically, hungry? How do I know when I'm full?*

EAT HOW MUCH YOU NEED—NOT HOW MUCH YOU *THINK* YOU SHOULD

A lot of factors probably contribute to the size of your meals: how much you put on your plate, what others around you are eating, and—if you're dieting—guilt about what you think you *should* do. But the truth is, only your body can tell you how much you need to consume. In mindful eating programs, "people think the idea is to get them to stop after one bite," says Dr. Lutes. "But we want you to eat what you want, but be mindful of it, actually enjoy it, and not feel guilty about it." In other words, if your body's signals are telling you to continue eating, then you have no reason to feel bad about doing so.

TRY TO BE MINDFUL *EVERY* TIME YOU EAT

You can eat mindfully at a buffet, a birthday party, or during Thanksgiving dinner. The key: Let your friends or family members do the talking at the start of the meal, buying you a few moments to take a mindful bite or two. Mini meditations are perhaps the easiest way to put this into practice. Before you eat, analyze your level of hunger and any emotions you're bringing to the table, and take a few deep breaths to help you focus on the food in front of you. (Some people find it helpful to close their eyes, but you don't have to.) About halfway through the meal, check in again, noticing the decrease in hunger and increase in fullness you're experiencing. This is a good time to answer the questions, "Do I really need to keep eating?" and "Am I satisfied?"

THREE TAKEAWAYS TO TRY TODAY

1. **Eat before you get hungry.** Eat at regular times. Don't skip meals or you'll set yourself up for intense cravings.

2. **Test your tongue.** Practice eating the way a food critic does: noting every flavor and texture.

3. **Always use a bowl or plate; never eat out of a box or bag.** You can't tell how much you're eating if you can't see it.

ASK THE LIFE STYLIST

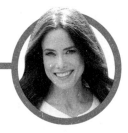

Keri Glassman, MS, RD, founder of
Nutritious Life, a nutrition practice
based in New York City

Q > I get hungry right before bed. Can I eat something?

A < Follow your hunger—not the clock—to decide when to
eat. That said, dehydration likes to pose as hunger, so first
drink a glass of water and wait 10 minutes. Still itching for a
nibble? If you do need a bite most evenings, add veggies (up
to 1 cup) to dinner. If that doesn't work, have 1 cup of skim
milk or ½ cup of cooked oatmeal before bed. Milk's tryptophan will help you doze off, and whole grains promote the
release of serotonin, which will help you relax.

Q > Is it okay if I cheat on my diet?

A < Most eating plans build in "cheat days," where you're
allowed to eat whatever you want, in whatever quantity you
want. The problem is, the notion of cheating attaches guilt to
eating, and that's the kind of thinking that predisposes you to
unhealthy patterns of consumption, like emotional eating or
even bingeing. That's why I prefer an "all things in moderation, all the time" approach. If you give yourself permission to
eat most of the foods you love—to say, "I can eat the dessert"—it enables you to control yourself, to have only half the
cupcake and feel totally satisfied. Very few foods are off-
limits in the 20 Pounds Younger program because we want
you to feel empowered, not deprived. Of course, choose as
healthfully as possible. So don't "cheat," just eat—mindfully,
and from a place of empowerment.

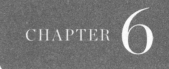
Ways to Eat "Clean" without Going Crazy / Ditch the Calorie Cutting and Enjoy

Don't wreck a sublime *chocolate experience* by feeling guilty.

–LORA BRODY, CHEF

HAVE YOU EVER TRIED TO STICK WITH SUPERSTRICT guidelines for eating that effectively eliminated all pleasure and flexibility from your diet? No doubt, pairing this hyperrestrictive approach with a low-calorie diet can and will cause you to lose weight. The question is, how long will your progress last? "People are very successful at losing weight initially. The issue is regain across time," says Lesley Lutes, PhD, an associate professor of psychology at East Carolina University. Low-calorie diets aren't sustainable over time, and they don't teach people how to live their lives differently, she says.

I think strict diets are just plain miserable, and I have a suspicion that you agree. I'm a hungry girl—and I *have* to eat at regular intervals, without a million rules telling me what I can't have. Research suggests that the restrictive rules people adopt are usually impossible to keep, so they set themselves up for failure. When psychologist Jean Kristeller, PhD, asks overweight clients how they *think* they should be eating, "they proceed to tell me a totally unrealistic eating pattern: Zero sweets. Maybe an egg and a piece of fruit for breakfast. A salad for lunch, then a piece of chicken with no skin and some steamed vegetables for dinner," she says. The grand total: about 1,000 calories per day. "They'd be starving," she says. "This is not maintainable for anybody who weighs more than about 90 pounds."

The idea that losing weight equals torturous sacrifice is perhaps one of the biggest food fallacies. The truth is, the relationship with eating that we wish we could all have—knowing when to stop and when to indulge without a shred of guilt—*is* possible and *can* help you lose weight. Psychologists have even coined a term for it: flexible restraint. "Weight management really

YO-YO? NO, NO

Why Up-and-Down Weight Fluctuations Hurt More Than Your Self-Image

Yo-yo dieting, where you lose a bunch of weight only to gain it back (and then some) a month later, is unhealthy. Here's why.

It could slow down your metabolism. New research in the *International Journal of Obesity* found that women whose weight fluctuated experienced a drop in resting energy expenditure—that is, the number of calories they burned while doing nothing. The researchers also found that when they regained lost weight, it was disproportionately in their arms and legs.

It may raise your risk of endometrial cancer. In a 2013 study in the *European Journal of Cancer,* women who lost and then regained weight one or more times were twice as likely to develop endometrial cancer. (The risk was especially high among those who'd been obese and who had also lost and gained 20-plus pounds at least once.)

It could make you hungrier. Yo-yo dieters tend to have higher levels of the appetite hormone ghrelin, according to a University of Washington study. The constant calorie sacrifice triggers a more forceful ghrelin response from your body.

should be about focusing on healthy foods that you like, rather than trying to stay away from foods that you like," says Katie Rickel, PhD, a clinical psychologist and weight-loss expert who works at a weight-management facility in Durham, North Carolina. Did you catch that? You should try to find good-for-you foods that you love and enjoy them, rather than obsessively condemning your favorite, but less-healthy, foods.

So instead of adopting rigid rules about what you can't have—no chocolate, cheese, or chips for this girl!—you need to create a set of flexible guidelines for what you *will* eat. In a *Journal of Consumer Research* study, women who said, "I don't eat that," rather than, "I can't eat that," were much more likely to adhere to their eating plans. "I can't" signals deprivation, which makes you more likely to cave, whereas "I don't" signals determination and empowerment, making your refusal more effective, according to one author of the study, Vanessa Patrick, PhD, of the University of Houston.

What do these easier-to-follow rules look like? As an example, Dr. Rickel often encourages clients to eat only at meals or planned snacks, but not in between. "That's a somewhat rigid guideline, but within that guideline, there is flexibility," she says. How can the two coexist? Simple: Her clients aren't saying "I must eat grilled chicken and asparagus" every night for dinner; they're just establishing a framework for when they will eat and then planning, say, to consume one source of lean protein, one vegetable, and a dash of healthy fat at each meal. "People do better when they have guidelines around what they're going to eat, rather than being very specific about what they're going to eat," she explains.

This also means you stop vilifying one food while glorifying another. You're simply determining which foods you want to focus on to meet your goals, then creating guidelines to help you fit those foods into your day. For example, you may decide that your daily afternoon snack will include fresh fruit. Then, to ensure your success, you plan ahead: You pack fruit, whether it's an apple or some cut-up cantaloupe, for work each day, or you make sure you have it on hand when you're out running errands.

You not only have flexibility in the fruit you choose, but you're also practicing forgiveness if you don't always follow that guideline 100 percent.

That's not to say that you should stray from your intended snack daily, but rather that if you're at a work conference, for example, and your food of choice isn't available, you survey the snack table and settle on an alternative that will satiate you. And you enjoy it, instead of beating yourself up over every bite, because flexibility is all part of your plan. "People are much more successful if they allow themselves to loosen up over a meal, or during a particular day, than if they try to white-knuckle through it," says Dr. Rickel. People who practice flexible restraint have been shown to be *less* prone to out-of-control eating and to have a lower average body mass index (BMI).

Compare that to a more rigid approach, where you treat rules like unbreakable commandments: In that case, if your one "allowed" food isn't available, you may feel totally thrown off and end up overdoing it, since you don't allow any room for a backup plan. "That's why rigid programs—those that cut out whole food groups or that allow you to eat only one particular food in one particular way—never really work. We're human beings, and human beings sometimes veer off path," says Dr. Rickel.

You don't have to give up indulgences—but you do have to pause before you plow through a bag of potato chips. "Ask yourself, 'Is this worth 800 calories to me?'" says Dr. Lutes. "If the answer is yes, then enjoy it, but be mindful about it." In other words, don't zone out because you feel so guilty that you can't stand to savor your food.

Why No Food Is Totally Off-Limits

The truth no one tells you: You can eat any food and still lose weight. The most nutrient-dense foods should, of course, be the stars of your eating plan (your body and mind will thank you), but you still have the freedom to indulge. You *can* have cake or a bowl of ice cream, or some chocolate. Anything. And you should no longer think about these foods as being "wrong." Instead, you should designate your "always" foods (the ones that make up the core of your diet) and your "sometimes" foods (the ones you eat on occasion).

Notice that there's no sense of rule breaking attached to this dietary dichotomy. "You're getting rid of the 'bad' foods and 'good' foods mentality," says Andrea Lieberstein, MPH, RD, a mindful eating instructor who directs Mind, Body, Spirit programs at Kaiser Permanente San Francisco. "If you want to have foods that are higher in fat and calories, the processed foods, then have them occasionally—give yourself permission to eat anything, but in smaller quantities, and savor it."

If you found yourself scoffing at that last part—smaller quantities, only a little bit—realize that this isn't about sacrifice. It's about tuning in to your taste buds and realizing when they're telling you, "I've had enough!" (Sometimes they don't speak loudly enough. You have to learn to listen.) "If we really pay attention to the foods we have a craving for, like cheese puffs, we may notice that they actually don't taste as good after a few bites," says Lieberstein. "The taste starts changing." As Brian Wansink, PhD, director of the Cornell University Food and Brand Lab, says, "It's a lot more liberating to say, 'I can eat whatever I want, whenever I want, as long as I know how much I actually want.'"

There's a danger to the deprivation that comes from the popular fasting techniques for weight loss, too. For some people, a fast can be empowering, offering an exercise in self-control. However, be aware that fasting can backfire. Studies have shown that even mild, short-term fasting can alter the foods people choose to eat, causing them to overcompensate by eating

INSTANT AGE ERASER

Upgrade Your Sweetener

Pure maple syrup has some sweet benefits, from immune-boosting zinc to antiaging antioxidants. In fact, University of Rhode Island researchers found that the sticky stuff contains 54 beneficial compounds—20 of which have known health benefits, such as natural anti-inflammatory and antibacterial properties. No matter how you pour it, syrup is still high in sugar, so drizzle sparingly, and use the kind that's tapped from a maple tree, not an imitation that grows on a cornstalk.

starches first—and lots of them—when they come off the fast. In a recent study in the *Archives of Internal Medicine,* two groups of college students were placed on either an 18-hour fast or no fast. At lunch after the 18 hours, all of the participants were allowed to eat from a buffet with their choice of two starches (dinner rolls and French fries), two proteins (chicken fingers and cheese), and two vegetables (carrots and green beans). Hidden scales recorded the amount of each food participants ate, and the researchers observed the order in which the foods were consumed. The study found that 47 percent of calories consumed during the meal came from whichever food the participants ate first. And what was the food the fasting participants reached for first? You guessed it: 75 percent of those who fasted started their next meal with the rolls, French fries, chicken fingers, or cheese, compared with 44 percent of the nonfasting participants.

Think about your own experience with dieting in the past. Have deprivation diets worked for you? There are three chocolate cupcakes on the kitchen table that look really tasty. What do you do? Deny yourself the dessert? Eat one or half of one? Eat two of them? Explore how you would feel after making each choice. There's a big difference between feelings of guilt and feelings of empowerment. The more you can make mindful choices that lead to empowerment, the more success you will find in reducing calories and eating healthier foods. In the next chapter, we'll learn simple ways that we can adapt our palates to make mindful eating even easier.

THREE TAKEAWAYS TO TRY TODAY

1. **Create guidelines,** but don't get too specific and restrictive. Rigid dieters often struggle to keep weight off.

2. **Rethink your food labels.** Just because it's called devil's food cake doesn't mean it's evil! Labeling foods as "sometimes" for indulgences and "always" for the good stuff will keep you on task better than quitting cold turkey.

3. **Make a choice.** Before you eat the cookie, think about how you'll feel afterward. Then if you decide you want it anyway, enjoy!

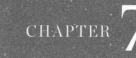

CHAPTER 7

A 4-Week Fix for Foodies/Evolve Your Palate and Learn Good Eating

REMEMBER WHEN YOU WERE A KID, AND THE CEREAL WITH the prize inside always seemed to taste the best? Of course, the sugar content was probably similar to that of every other brightly colored box, but the little trinket buried among the rice puffs tricked your brain into preferring that brand. Or maybe it was the cute character who sold you on that particular cereal: In a 2010 Yale University study, kids tended to think that foods with recognizable characters on the packaging tasted better.

Of course, you're no longer 6 years old and swayed by cartoon animals on cereal boxes. But you *do* probably have some ingrained ideas about which foods you like—and which ones you despise. Research suggests that, from birth, we tend to prefer sweet and salty foods to bitter and sour ones, which explains toddlers' disdain for vegetables and tart fruits. Once upon a time, this was adaptive, since in the days of early man, sweetness usually signaled nutritional value and bitterness could indicate toxicity, say University of California–Santa Barbara scientists. The problem is, not all bitter foods are truly toxic. Green vegetables in particular often have bitter flavors and are therefore less palatable.

Fortunately, exposure may shape our palates as much as—if not more than—our inborn predispositions. "The more you eat a food, the more you want it, whether it's unhealthy or healthy. It's sort of like flavor memory," says Dawn Jackson Blatner, RD, a nutrition consultant for the Chicago Cubs. Before you were even born, you were exposed to the flavors of the foods your mother ate, and as an infant, you were introduced to new tastes through breast milk or formula.

What your parents piled on your plate further expanded—or limited—the foods your palate favors. "When children grow up in India, they tolerate eating very spicy curries," says Blatner. "But if children are only exposed to chicken nuggets, they develop a flavor profile for bland fried foods." This even applies to veggies, the most stereotypically hated foods among kids: In a study in the journal *Appetite,* the more frequently children were offered vegetables, the more they reported liking them. This, the study authors say, is evidence that simple exposure may be the key to developing a taste for new foods, even bitter ones.

There's also proof of this in the animal kingdom: Like humans, fruit flies tend to reject bitter foods. But in a University of California study, researchers fed the winged insects camphor—a bitter-tasting but nontoxic chemical—and after a while, the flies began to consume it willingly. Another study found that as rats age, they become less averse to bitter flavors; similarly, in humans, age seems to decrease our taste for sweets. "Our taste buds, whether you're a young child or an adult set in your ways, absolutely have the ability to change," Blatner says. It's adaptive for our palates to be flexible: If our tastes were fixed, we would have been wiped out in times of famine, when only a select few foods were available—especially if they were foods we didn't particularly like.

INSTANT AGE ERASER

Go Greek

Switch from regular fruit yogurt, which has 1.78 times the age-adding refined sugar as Greek yogurt with fresh fruit. Since even fresh fruit can be high in sugar content, you can trim calories further by skipping the fruit and choosing plain full-fat Greek yogurt with just a drizzle of pure maple syrup or honey for flavor.

I call this "evolving your palate," and I can personally attest to the truth of this phenomenon. Back in my candy-loving days, I wanted—and even thought I needed—a sizable dose of sugar after every meal, no matter how full I was. But as I shifted my focus to whole foods, I found that not only had this yearning for sugar dissipated, but also that my taste buds could no longer tolerate the saccharine sweetness they once craved. Same goes for juices: I would have once grimaced at a green drink—liquefied spinach, really?—but I now see veggie-based juices as sustenance. Sunshine, even; a bright spot in my day. As weird as this may sound, the truly unnatural thing is eating highly processed foods; we're built to fuel up on fruits, vegetables, and lean protein, not sugary substitutes concocted in a laboratory.

Evolving Your Palate: Your Step-by-Step Plan

If you've spent years eating processed foods, you've probably developed a taste for supersweet *and* highly salty foods, the most pleasant components in the taste palate. You may even feel the urge to eat one after the other: cheesy chips followed by chocolate ice cream, then back to salty with a handful of pretzels. Still, you probably have a preference, favoring either sweet or salty foods, and you could even be addicted.

But just because that's what you like *now* doesn't mean you have to be a sweet-and-salty fiend for life. If you deliberately expose your palate to less-sugary or less-salty foods, you'll eventually find your preferences changing. For example, though a big slab of milk chocolate may have once been your go-to treat, you may find that it's simply too sugary and that a few squares of dark chocolate quiets your sweet tooth.

Don't worry, we're not going to ask you to give up your favorite munchies cold turkey. And keep in mind, these steps aren't necessary for everybody—some of you may be able to eat salty or sugary foods on occasion with no problem, and your palate may naturally evolve away from those foods as you start to eat healthier ones. But if you have consistent cravings for either type of snack, try to slowly retrain your palate to prefer less-sweet or less-salty indulgences. It takes about a month, but it's easy to do. By the end, you won't even miss the processed foods of your past.

IF YOU HAVE A SWEET TOOTH . . .

WEEK 1: *Replace One Sugary Beverage with Water or Unsweetened Iced Tea Daily*

Most people are well aware that soda is a weight-gain culprit, but did you know that fruit juice isn't exactly a solid pick either? In a Harris Interactive poll, nearly half of Americans said they think juice is healthy. But the fact is, most bottles are filled with little more than sugar, without any of the redeeming fiber you'll find in actual fruit. So make it your mission to substitute water or tea for one additional sugary beverage each day until you've eliminated the stuff entirely. You may be surprised at how quickly this has an impact on the number you see on the scale. In one study, women who replaced juice and soda with water dropped 3 pounds more than dieters who didn't. (And those who downed more than four glasses of water each day lost an extra 2 pounds.)

WEEK 2: *Cut Out Artificial Sweeteners*

Wait, isn't sugar—not its artificial substitutes—the enemy? Although sugar replacements might seem like an easy way around your sweet tooth—they're calorie-free!—they are actually significantly sweeter than sugar. (Aspartame, for example, is up to 220 times sweeter than the real stuff!) As a result, artificial sweeteners can increase your preference for sweetness and trigger sugar cravings, according to the *Yale Journal of Biology and Medicine*. A recent study from the University of North Carolina–Chapel Hill found that diet-soda drinkers ate more desserts and bread—hello, empty carbs!—than people who sipped the regular stuff. "Substitutes may not signal the same satiety hormones as sugar, making it easier to overeat," says Lona Sandon, RD, an assistant professor of nutrition at the University of Texas–Southwestern.

Where do these sugar stand-ins hide? You'll find them in diet soda,

HATE DARK CHOCOLATE? YOU CAN CHANGE THAT!

People who favor dark chocolate are 2.5 times more tolerant of bitter flavors, according to a 2012 study in the *Journal of Food Science*. But if you're a milk chocolate fiend, you may just need to train your palate to accept the darker stuff.

You could, of course, just gradually increase the percentage of cacao—the ingredient actually derived from the cocoa bean—in the bars you buy, slowly shifting from 30 percent to 50 percent to 80 or 90 percent. But nutritionist Dawn Jackson Blatner, RD, suggests a different approach: Use a cheese grater to create dark chocolate shavings—go for the 80 to 90 percent cacao stuff—and then pair them with a fruit you like, such as sliced strawberries, bananas, or raspberries. "After a week of having fruit and superdark chocolate, you not only establish exposure, but you also become more likely to enjoy dark chocolate even on its own," she says. "For some people, this might take 4 days, and for others, 14. But 10 days of exposure is average."

sugar-free packaged foods, reduced-calorie yogurts, and canned fruit. You can also just scan the ingredients list for acesulfame-K, stevia, sucralose (Splenda), aspartame (Equal, NutraSweet), and saccharin (Sweet'N Low)—all common zero-calorie sweeteners. And, of course, this means no more adding little packets of sugar substitutes to your coffee.

WEEK 3: *Avoid Packaged and Processed Foods with Added Sugars*

There are good-for-you natural sugars, like those found in fruit, and then there are added sugars, the ones that don't naturally occur in food but that manufacturers add for flavor. Unfortunately, detecting sugar in packaged foods is not always as simple as scanning for it in the ingredients panel. Sugar hides in places you wouldn't expect because it's cheap to produce, tasty, and addictive. You'll find it in everything from salad dressing to pasta sauces.

So before you buy a packaged food, check for added sugar pseudonyms: barley-malt syrup, brown rice syrup, high-fructose corn syrup, fructose, galactose, glucose, maltodextrin, molasses, sorghum, sucrose, and turbinado. This is the simplest way to clean up any diet. If you already have sugar-laden packaged foods at home, consider removing one item each day until your refrigerator and pantry are clear.

WEEK 4: *Make Two of Your Meals at Home Each Day—Without Adding Any Sugar*

Even the most savory of restaurant dishes can be sugar bombs. And the scary part is that you may have no idea, since most of us assume a pasta dish isn't coated in sugar. That's one reason people take in 36 percent more calories at restaurants compared to when they dine at home. "One of the biggest signs of unhealthy eating habits is an unused kitchen," says dietitian Amy Baertschi, RD. So bring out your inner chef and lean on herbs and spices, not sugar, for flavor.

IF YOU CRAVE SALTY FOODS . . .

Our tongues are specially designed to detect sodium, and our bodies require sodium to survive. But why do we start seeking out the stuff? Force of habit may actually be more to blame than a salt addiction, according to a study

---

INSTANT AGE ERASER

Rosemary

Food flavorer *and* sight saver? A compound in rosemary called carnosic acid could reduce your risk for age-related macular degeneration, the most common cause of vision loss in the United States, according to a study in the journal *Investigative Ophthalmology and Visual Science*. Carnosic acid may protect retinal cells from the deterioration and toxicity caused by free radicals.

review in *Neuroscience and Biobehavioral Reviews*. The scientists point out that people often salt their food before they've even tasted it, suggesting that we're often on autopilot when we pick up the saltshaker; it's almost like the muscle memory you develop after performing an exercise over and over again. What that means is that to break your salt habit, you may just need to change your habits, and your taste buds will follow suit.

WEEK 1: *Rid Your Pantry of Highly Processed Snacks*

How do we define "highly processed"? Keri Glassman, MS, RD, founder of Nutritious Life, a nutrition practice based in New York City, says there are many ways: long shelf life, number of ingredients, number of artificial ingredients, etc. Ask yourself, "Is it real food?" One of the key telltale signs of highly processed food, she says, is sodium content above 140 milligrams per serving. (This is a threshold even the FDA abides by: In order to be labeled "low sodium," soups must contain 140 milligrams of sodium or less per serving.) And make sure to check nutritional panels of foods you don't suspect are super salty, too: A recent Centers for Disease Control and Prevention (CDC) report revealed that bread, cold cuts, and cheese are top sources of salt in the American diet—even more so than savory snacks like chips, popcorn, and pretzels.

WEEK 2: *Replace One Prepackaged Snack with Fresh Fruit or Vegetables Each Day*

Even if you've cleared out the junk from your pantry, you may still be tempted by salty vending-machine snacks or convenience-store foods. Your goal: Gradually replace these processed snacks with whole-food options. "Continue to replace one prepackaged snack with fresh fruits or vegetables per day until all snacks are fresh," says Glassman. "I don't mind when people use a little bit of sea salt when cooking. It's the packaged, processed foods that are the worst." (Restaurant food is also bad, so restrain yourself from using the saltshaker when dining out.)

WEEK 3: *Toss Out Your Saltshaker*

This isn't a permanent move! You just need to train your taste buds not to depend so much on salt for pleasure. "When people cut salt out of their diet, and then it is reintroduced, they can use lower levels of salt," says Lucy Donaldson, PhD, associate professor of physiology at the University of Nottingham, in England. "And they often prefer lower levels, even if they previously had high salt intake." After a couple weeks, bring back the saltshaker, but make a point of using it only after you've tasted your food. You may find that you don't need it after all.

ARE YOU A SUPERTASTER?

If you have a serious sweet tooth, you may partly have your genetics to blame, since taste inclinations are coded in our DNA. A study published in *Physiology and Behavior* found that up to 45 percent of our food preferences are determined by genetics. Among the things controlled by biology is the number of taste buds you have, and some people have anywhere from 10 to 100 times more than average. That, in combination with genes that influence what you taste, could make you especially sensitive to the flavors of foods— or what food scientists call a "supertaster." This palate quirk, when coupled with a sweet tooth, may lead you to shun some veggies and favor desserts (not a good thing, by the way). Being finicky about what you eat is one sign that you may be a supertaster. But there's also a more scientific way to determine whether you have an exaggerated sense of taste, and it makes a great party trick: Simply squeeze one drop of blue food coloring onto your tongue, near the tip. Then place a round reinforcement sticker (the kind meant to keep holes in loose-leaf paper from tearing) over the dye, and count the number of fungiform papillae (the little bumps on your tongue that contain your taste buds) within the circle. See more than 30? That means you're a supertaster.

WEEK 4: *Incorporate Herbs and Spices into as Many Meals as Possible*

Once you've brought back salt, start experimenting with herbs and spices when you're cooking. "That way, you're less likely to go back to the salt-shaker," says Glassman. Read: If you learn to add flavor in other ways, you won't need to depend on salt to stimulate your taste buds—and you'll find it easier to resist the urge to sprinkle the stuff liberally on every meal you eat.

THREE TAKEAWAYS TO TRY TODAY

1. **Cut your juice with water** or, if you must drink it straight, have only a tiny glass. Orange and apple juices qualify as unhealthy due to the number of calories from sugar they contain.

2. **Drop cold cuts from your diet to dramatically reduce your sodium intake.** Deli meats and cheeses are loaded with salt.

3. **Reduce your daily calorie consumption simply by cooking a meal at home** instead of eating at a restaurant.

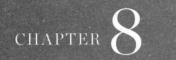

CHAPTER 8

The 20 Pounds Younger Eating Plan/Swap the Empty Calories for Meals That Are Clean and Lean

MINDFUL EATING WORKS. IF YOU CAN CONDITION YOURSELF to pause and consider your food choice before you commit your tongue, you have learned a great secret of weight loss and maintenance. But it's not the only one. Having a solid plan that becomes second nature to you can help a great deal. In fact, for some people, a written plan can do wonders for keeping strategies and goals at the front of their minds and for controlling the number of calories they consume.

See, calories *do* count to a certain degree. A meta-analysis of dozens of nutrition studies by Brazilian researchers found that reducing calorie intake accounts for 75 percent of weight loss, versus 25 percent from exercise. You've heard that before? It's real. It's true. And it's great news for those of you who don't like to sweat! But that doesn't mean you have to *count* calories, something that many women find time-consuming, difficult, and a real bummer. Plus, can you think of any easier way to toss a wet napkin on a great meal?

Psychologist Jean Kristeller, PhD, has a different take on the whole calorie-counting thing. She suggests a vocabulary change, switching the word calories with a new term: food energy. (You don't actually have to say it in public!) This change in terminology helps you view meals in terms of the fuel they provide—and whether it's a slow-burning, energy-efficient fuel or a fast-burning, hungry-in-an-hour kind. There's a big difference.

Dietitian Keri Glassman agrees that calories are just one measure of a food's merit. "Ingredients and quality matter the most," she says. "Your body processes nutrients differently." In other words, your system will respond very differently to a 400-calorie meal built on lean protein and complex carbs than it would to a 400-calorie bowl of pudding. Calories aren't as important as what's inside the food: the macronutrients, protein, carbohydrates, and fat; and the vitamins, minerals, and fiber—not to mention what hopefully is *not* there, namely preservatives and other chemicals.

If you dislike calorie counting, you're in luck. Portion control will take care of reducing calories. Practicing portion control is more about providing your body with the amount of food it needs than staying within a prescribed number of calories. So instead of saying, "I can have 200 calories' worth of fish," you start with a 4-ounce portion—but with the options of (1) not cleaning your plate or (2) dishing out a little more if your body tells you to. You might find you need only 3 ounces, or you might be hungrier, so you need 5 ounces. "You have that starting place—the 4-ounce portion—and then from there you learn to listen to your body and have confidence in making those choices to have a little bit more or a little bit less," says Glassman. As a food lover, I've found this approach a lot easier to manage.

As I mentioned, the other way to help make portion control and food choices easier is to ensure that you're getting the right mix of food types by using a physical "cheat sheet," or as I like to call it, an "Eat Sheet." Hell, call it the "Cut the Crappy Food Cue Card" if that works for you, because that's exactly what it does. It's like a to-do list for your daily diet—an easy way to remember the principal guidelines of the eating plan that Glassman has designed for us. Follow it, and you'll automatically elbow out the sugar-and-salt-laden, highly processed foods that lead to weight gain, ensuring that you eat the cleanest antifat, antistress, antioxidant, antiaging foods you can.

{The Eat Sheet}

Check off these daily do's to erase pounds and years from your figure.

☐☐ **Drink a glass** of water with lemon before breakfast.

☐ **Eat breakfast** within 90 minutes of waking.

☐☐☐ Do a **mini meditation** before each meal.

☐☐ Eat **two servings of greens** per day.

☐☐☐ Include **one mood-boosting nutrient** in every meal.

☐☐☐ Eat **one protein and/or fat** at every meal.

☐ Make **legumes, vegetables, or ancient grains** (see this chapter for a complete list) your primary sources of complex carbohydrates.

☐☐ Eat **two snacks** per day containing protein, fat, and/or fiber.

 Fill (and refill) a 16-ounce water bottle with **water** and sip from it all day. Goal: eight full bottles.

The Eat Sheet Explained

Let's break down these Eat Sheet guidelines and explore what makes them so effective at turning back the clock.

☑ DRINK A GLASS OF WATER WITH LEMON BEFORE BREAKFAST.

Water fills you up and helps keep your metabolism running on high—but there's also a psychological reason to grab a glass: "You're signaling to yourself that you're starting the day off healthy, telling yourself, 'I'm going to be good to my body today,'" says Glassman. So fill up a big glass, add a slice of lemon, and guzzle it before or with your breakfast. Lemon water cleanses the liver, your body's main fat-burning organ. Another great option: Squeeze the juice of half a lemon into a mug of warm water. Warm lemon water promotes peristalsis, the contraction of bowel muscles that keeps waste moving along the digestive tract for elimination. You'll start your day good to go.

☑ EAT BREAKFAST WITHIN 90 MINUTES OF WAKING.

When you wake up after a full night's sleep, your body is in fasting mode. Without food for 8 or so hours, your metabolism has slowed down, so you need to rev it up again with breakfast. You may notice less moodiness throughout the day if you do: There's evidence that people who eat breakfast—and we're not talking a pastry—have more consistent moods and are less likely to battle severe depression. And many, many studies have revealed that breakfast eaters weigh less, keep weight off longer, and reduce their risks of both obesity and diabetes relative to people who always skip breakfast. It's well documented.

☑ DO A MINI MEDITATION BEFORE EACH MEAL.

If you learn to listen to your body, you may find that portion control happens naturally—because, let's be honest, nobody *really* needs a 2-pound hamburger or an extra-large sweet tea. Mini meditations—simply being mindful as you take a few deep breaths before eating and noticing your hunger level, thoughts, and emotions—can tune you in to your internal experience. The outcome: You'll know when to put down the fork, because you'll know when you're no longer hungry. For specific instructions, see Chapter 4.

☑ EAT TWO SERVINGS OF GREENS PER DAY.

Green vegetables are nutritional powerhouses, chock-full of disease-fighting antioxidants, fiber, and water to fill you up, and they also contain a bevy of essential vitamins and minerals. Specifically, "leafy greens are typically low on the glycemic index, high in phytonutrients, fiber, and vitamins, and have innumerable health benefits—cardioprotective qualities, cholesterol-lowering benefits, and anticancer properties," says Glassman. In a study of carb-conscious dieters, the biggest weight losers ate four servings of non-starchy vegetables—that includes both leafy and nonleafy greens—per day. Nonleafy greens are cool, too. In fact, broccoli, artichoke, and asparagus—all nonleafy greens—tend to be more hearty and satisfying than leafy greens.

Portion size? Go wild. Eat as much as you like because these foods are nutrient dense and low in calories.

The Greens Team

LEAFY

> Beet greens

> Bok choy

> Collard greens

> Kale

> Mustard greens

> Romaine lettuce

> Spinach

> Swiss chard

> Turnip greens

NONLEAFY

> Artichoke

> Asparagus

> Broccoli

> Brussels sprouts

> Celery

> Cucumber

☑ INCLUDE ONE MOOD-BOOSTING NUTRIENT IN EVERY MEAL.

Certain nutrients and vitamins influence the chemical balance of your brain to lift your spirits and even ward off depression. By making a conscious effort to get a bit of these foods into every main meal, you'll prime your brain with added firepower against emotional eating. There are lots of them, so it should be easy to do this without driving yourself bonkers. Let's take a look at the main mood-boosting nutrients, how they perform their feel-good magic, and where to find them. Try a variety of mood boosters and make an effort to have one every time you eat.

OMEGA-3 FATTY ACIDS. By now, we've all heard about the merits of incorporating fish oils in your diet thanks to the heart-helping, brain-preserving, inflammation-fighting, flab-blasting abilities of the omega-3s they contain. These good-for-you fats have the power to stabilize your

YOUR DAILY DOSE OF OMEGA-3s

Fish haters, fear not: You can load up on omega-3 fatty acids in capsule form—although, keep in mind, fish aren't the only source of these good fats (see the next page). If you prefer to pop a pill, look for the letters EPA and DHA on the label; this indicates the presence of two highly unsaturated essential fatty acids that play important roles in our bodies. Choose a fish oil supplement with about 500 milligrams each of EPA and DHA, such as those by Nordic Naturals and Coromega. Hate the fishy burps? Freeze your capsules and take them with meals to avoid this nasty side effect.

PICK YOUR PORTION

Mood Foods

Ancient grains: ⅓ to
½ cup cooked

Beans and legumes:
½ cup

Cantaloupe, papaya,
pineapple, strawberries:
1 cup cubes or berries

Grapefruit: ½ medium

Kiwifruit, oranges: 1 small

Red-skinned potatoes:
½ cup diced

Steel-cut or old-fashioned
oats: ⅓ cup cooked

Sweet potatoes: ½ small

Nonstarchy vegetables:
Eat as much as you want!

mood, too—an effect that may be especially pronounced in women, research suggests.

The antidepressant benefit of omega-3s makes sense when you consider the biology of your brain, the central command center for your moods. "Sixty percent of the brain is fat," says Elizabeth Somer, MA, RD, author of *Food & Mood.* According to French researchers, omega-3s make up about a tenth of that fat, so it's no surprise that these fatty acids play a critical role in mental health. "The more fluid and flexible the brain cells, the less likely you are to battle depression down the road," says Somer. "And the most fluid and flexible fats are omega-3s, so when given the chance, our brains preferentially take up omega-3s to build brain cells."

Not all omega-3s are created equal, though. The best depression fighter is docosahexaenoic acid (DHA), one of the fatty acids found in fish like salmon and sardines. Up to 97 percent of the omega-3s in your brain are DHA. However, alpha-linolenic acid (ALA), the omega-3 found in plants, still has a place in your mood-boosting plan. "ALA has to be converted to DHA in your body," says Glassman. And unfortunately, it's not a one-to-one conversion. "You're not getting as much, but that's not to say these foods, especially eaten regularly, aren't contributing," she says.

Omega-3-Rich Foods

> Chia seeds

> Flaxseeds

> Salmon

> Sardines (Pacific)

> Soybeans (non-GMO)

> Walnuts

COMPLEX CARBOHYDRATES. These slow-burning starches qualify as mood-boosting foods because of how they influence the amino acid tryptophan, which is the precursor to the mood-regulating, appetite-suppressing brain chemical serotonin. Not to get too technical here, but tryptophan is a pretty bulky molecule that has some difficulty getting into your brain without help. That's why a turkey drumstick alone isn't exactly going to make your day. But if you eat the tryptophan-rich protein with some complex carbohydrates, the surge of insulin you get from the carbs shuttles the competing amino acids out of your bloodstream, leaving tryptophan a clear path through the blood-brain barrier, where it can be converted into serotonin and give your mood a boost. You need only a 30-gram dose of carbs—the amount found in a little more than $\frac{1}{2}$ cup of cooked brown rice—to experience the uplifting effect.

There's no need to count carb grams, though. If you eat a balanced diet that includes complex carbs—like ancient grains, oatmeal, and potatoes—you'll keep your ratio of tryptophan to other amino acids at a more optimal level, compared to if you followed a high-protein diet alone. That means your serotonin levels will be less likely to fall into the red, says Glassman.

Serotonin-Boosting Complex Carbs

> Ancient grains (see page 90 for a complete list)

> Red-skinned potatoes

> Steel-cut or old-fashioned oats

> Sweet potatoes

VITAMIN C. Remember the stress hormone cortisol? Vitamin C is your remedy. By including vitamin C–rich food in your meals, you will help your body combat stress, high blood pressure, and other responses to psychological tension while boosting your mood. And most of the vegetable sources of C on the list below are also good sources of complex carbs, so they'll do double-duty.

Vitamin C–Rich Foods

> Bell peppers
> Bok choy
> Broccoli
> Brussels sprouts
> Cabbage
> Cantaloupe
> Cauliflower
> Grapefruit
> Kale
> Kiwifruit
> Oranges
> Papaya
> Pineapple
> Strawberries
> Turnip greens

FOLIC ACID. A lack of folate could explain why you feel like you're in a funk. "Depressed people often have lower levels of this nutrient in their bodies," says Glassman. In fact, by some estimates, one-third of depressed people have a folate shortage, and those with the greatest deficiency tend to be the most melancholy (and are the least responsive to antidepressants), according to a study review in the *British Medical Journal*. One possible reason: Folic acid contributes to the production of neurotransmitters, including mood-regulating serotonin.

Folate-Rich Foods

> Asparagus
> Black beans
> Broccoli
> Brussels sprouts
> Chickpeas
> Garbanzo beans
> Kidney beans
> Lentils

> Navy beans

> Oranges

> Pinto beans

> Spinach

> Tomato juice

☑ EAT ONE PROTEIN AND/OR FAT AT EVERY MEAL.

Both macronutrients are satisfying belly fillers. Eating them will quell your hunger fast, so make one or both part of every main meal.

FATS. News flash: Eating fat will *not* make you fat. In fact, it's one of the easiest ways to make your meals more filling and flavorful—and may even help you burn fat, says Glassman. As long as your portions are reasonable—you don't need much fat to ramp up the fullness factor—your waistline won't complain. Another reason fat isn't the enemy: It helps your body utilize vitamins A, D, E, and K. "Fat in a salad dressing is going to help you absorb the good stuff in the greens," says Glassman.

By now, you've probably heard that some fats are "bad" and others are "good." But really, the only fats you want to steer clear of entirely are manmade trans fats (aka hydrogenated or partially hydrogenated oils), which have been linked to heart disease and obesity. But the rest are fair game! Make monounsaturated fats (found in olive oil and nuts) and polyunsaturated fats

---

PICK YOUR PORTION

Avocado: ¼ medium

Organic pasture butter: 2 teaspoons

Coconut: 1 tablespoon

Nuts: about 10

Nut butter: 2 teaspoons

Olives: 12

Oils: 2 teaspoons

Seeds: 2 tablespoons

(found in fatty fish and some nuts and seeds) a priority, since these have the most health benefits.

You can even work in a little bit of saturated fat by adding a pat of organic butter to your veggies or by incorporating a little shredded coconut into a smoothie, for example. "There is some research suggesting that saturated fats—the real kind found in meat and dairy—can have a beneficial role in heart health," says Glassman. "A little bit might actually do something good for you. So you can have a little butter on you sweet potato if that's what you're craving." Coconut contains medium-chain triglycerides, a type of saturated fat with different benefits from the kind in meat and butter. This type of fat has specifically been linked to improved cholesterol and even fat burning.

Good-Fat Foods

> Avocado

> Coconut

> Nut and seed butters: almond, cashew, coconut, hazelnut, peanut, pistachio, sunflower seed

> Nuts: almonds, Brazil nuts, cashews, hazelnuts, peanuts, pecans, pine nuts, pistachios, walnuts

> Oils: coconut, flaxseed, grapeseed, hempseed, olive, walnut

> Olives

> Organic pasture butter

> Seeds: chia, hemp, pumpkin

PROTEIN. Protein is one of the best get-lean nutrients you can eat, and its slimming effects kick in the second you start chewing by instantly boosting your satisfaction *and* your calorie burning. Compared to carbs or fat, your body expends significantly more calories breaking down protein: For every 100 calories of protein you take in, you burn 23 during digestion. Plus, it can take up to 4 hours to digest, so you feel fuller longer. "Lean protein helps keep you satisfied and helps you build and repair muscle," says Glassman. "It's also important for maintaining and making hormones."

PICK YOUR PORTION

Protein

Beans: ½ cup

Eggs: 1 medium

Greek yogurt: 6 ounces

Firm tofu: 4 ounces

Meat, poultry, and fish: 4 to 6 ounces (let your hunger be your guide)

Seeds: 2 tablespoons

Protein-Rich Foods

- Albacore tuna
- Black beans
- Chicken (skinless, white or dark)
- Chickpeas
- Cod
- Eggs
- Firm tofu
- Grass-fed beef
- Greek yogurt (full-fat)

- Hemp seeds
- Kidney beans
- Lentils
- Lima beans
- Pinto beans
- Pork loin
- Salmon (freshwater, coho)
- Sardines (Pacific)
- Turkey

☑ **MAKE LEGUMES, VEGETABLES, OR ANCIENT GRAINS YOUR PRIMARY SOURCES OF COMPLEX CARBOHYDRATES.**

Carbs have gotten a bad rap, thanks to the overly processed—and nutrient-stripped—kinds found in white breads and other baked goods. But the truth is, your body needs carbohydrates for energy, and the good kind can actually help keep your waistline in check: A recent study in the

American Journal of Clinical Nutrition found that people who consumed the most whole grains had 17 percent less belly fat than those who ate the least. Unlike processed carbs, whole grains include the entire plant seed: the germ, bran, and endosperm—which means that all of their natural fiber is intact. That equals a full belly for you.

Why the focus on ancient grains? "You'll get carbs in other places in your diet—yogurt, fruits, and vegetables—but ancient grains are another way to get unprocessed carbs," says Glassman. "They are the least processed of all the grains." In other words, while 100 percent whole wheat bread is undoubtedly a better choice than white, it's still more processed than, say, a bowl of quinoa. And less processing may equal a brighter mood: Scientists from New Zealand say that complex carbs seem to lift people's spirits, while simple carbs breed a bad mood. Most ancient grains may be unfamiliar to you, so here's an introduction to some of my favorites.

Amaranth

TASTE: Slightly sweet, yet peppery

BENEFIT: This gluten-free grain is approximately 14 percent protein (and it's the complete kind, like you'll find in animal products), making it one of the most filling grains on the shelf. It's also one of the few grains that contains vitamin C.

PERFECT IT: Boil amaranth for 15 to 20 minutes—and don't skimp on the water! For every cup of amaranth, use about 6 cups of water.

Barley

TASTE: Slightly nutty

BENEFIT: Barley contains more fiber than any other whole grain. It's especially high in cholesterol-lowering beta-glucan, a type of fiber also found in oats.

PERFECT IT: Since barley can take up to an hour to cook, try whipping up a big batch and eating it throughout the week.

Ancient Grains
All ancient grains: ⅓ to ½ cup cooked

Buckwheat

TASTE: Robust, nutty

BENEFIT: Although not technically a grain—buckwheat is actually a cousin of rhubarb—its flavor and grainlike appearance earn it a spot among the ancient grains. Buckwheat is rich in rutin (a flavonoid that has potent antioxidant properties) and heart-healthy magnesium. Plus, it's gluten-free!

PERFECT IT: Make sure to follow the package instructions to toast buckwheat in a skillet until it's dry. Otherwise, it may swell up and turn into a thick, unsavory mass.

Bulgur

TASTE: Mild, nutty

BENEFIT: Bulgur is loaded with the mineral magnesium. It cooks quickly, making it a nutritious fast food.

PERFECT IT: This grain usually comes precooked, so just heat it up in boiling water for 20 to 25 minutes. Use about 2 cups of water per cup of bulgur.

Farro

TASTE: Warm, nutty, slightly sweet

BENEFIT: A staple for ancient Egyptians and modern-day Italians alike, farro has more fiber and protein than brown rice, plus a dose of calcium and iron. (Note: Make sure the package says "whole farro" to ensure that you're buying an unprocessed variety.)

PERFECT IT: Check the package before preparing farro, because some varieties require presoaking. When you're ready to cook it, use about 2 quarts of water per cup of farro. Expect it to double in volume during cooking.

Kamut

TASTE: Rich, buttery

BENEFIT: This heirloom grain has more protein and vitamin E than wheat. Only buy a box if it says "whole kamut" to guarantee you're getting the whole grain form.

PERFECT IT: Soak kamut overnight, then boil it, using about 3 cups of water per cup of the grain. Let it simmer for 30 to 40 minutes.

Millet

TASTE: Mildly sweet, delicately nutty

BENEFIT: This tiny grain is rarely eaten in the United States (except by birds), but it should be: Half a cup contains 38 milligrams of magnesium, plus 54 milligrams of potassium.

PERFECT IT: Use about $2\frac{1}{2}$ cups of water per cup of millet. Allow it to simmer for 13 to 18 minutes.

Quinoa

TASTE: Similar to wheat

BENEFIT: This round, gluten-free seed from a grainlike crop won't spike your blood sugar, and it's a complete protein, meaning it contains all nine essential amino acids. For an extra antioxidant boost, opt for red quinoa.

PERFECT IT: Be sure to rinse well because the tiny seeds have a bitter coating that needs to be rinsed off. Boil quinoa for 15 minutes, using 2 cups of water per cup of quinoa, then fluff it with a fork before serving.

Spelt

TASTE: Nutty

BENEFIT: It can easily stand in for wheat—a good thing, since spelt is higher in protein. Warning: Not all spelt is whole grain, so make sure the ingredients list says "whole spelt."

PERFECT IT: Use 3½ cups of water per cup of spelt. Bring it to a boil, reduce the heat, and then simmer for about 90 minutes.

Teff

TASTE: Sweet, molasses-like

BENEFIT: Teff is loaded with iron and leads the whole grain pack in terms of calcium content.

PERFECT IT: For creamy teff, cook 1 cup of the grain in 3 cups of water for 20 minutes.

Wheat berries

TASTE: Sweet, nutty, complex

BENEFIT: Wheat berries are a reliable source of protein, fiber, and iron. Look for the whole, not pearled, variety to ensure that you're really getting the whole grain.

PERFECT IT: Soak your wheat berries overnight, then cook them for 45 to 60 minutes, using 4 cups of water per cup of berries.

☑ EAT TWO SNACKS A DAY CONTAINING PROTEIN, FAT, AND/OR FIBER.

The logic behind snacking is nothing more than this: A calorie infusion between meals keeps your blood sugar stable and hunger under control so you don't feel famished come mealtime and overeat, or start binge eating before a meal because your blood sugar is low. In a Harvard University study, people who regularly munched on nuts—a snack that contains healthy fats and protein—were less likely to gain weight over time than those who didn't consume them as often. Of course, not all snacks are created equal—eating a handful of refined-carb crackers isn't going to do much for your body in terms of holding you over between meals. So what *will* keep your belly happy? "Snacks that contain protein, fat, and fiber keep you full and satisfied," says Glassman. "You go into your next meal without being ravenous, so you're more likely to make good decisions." Your snacks should fall in the 150- to 200-calorie range, depending on how hungry you are. However, if you prefer to simply practice portion control—which we suggest—instead of counting calories, try these proven hunger-busting snack combos.

> Sliced carrots + 10 raw almonds

> Cherry tomatoes + 1 ounce feta cheese + balsamic vinegar

> 6 ounces full-fat Greek yogurt + cinnamon + 1 tablespoon chia seeds

> 1 slice sprouted grain toast + 2 teaspoons natural peanut butter + nutmeg

> 12 raw pecans + 2 dried apricots + 2 tablespoons hummus + red and yellow pepper slices

> 2 fiber-rich crackers + 2 teaspoons natural nut butter + ½ teaspoon honey

> ⅓ cup cooked quinoa + 1 tablespoon guacamole

☑ DRINK EIGHT 16-OUNCE BOTTLES OF WATER PER DAY.

It sounds like a lot, but it's really not that hard if you keep that tumbler filled, sip regularly, and take it wherever you go. Oh, and you will *go* more often, for sure. But water works in the weight-loss game, studies show. Water fills your belly so you're not as hungry. (In fact, hunger is often simply a dehydration cue that you read the wrong way.) It helps with digestion. Well-hydrated skin looks younger. Even the frequent trips to the ladies' room burn a few extra calories. And if you think there is no way you could possibly drink that much H_2O, consider that the coffee, tea, and unsweetened iced tea that you drink every day count toward you water quota.

Make water work harder: Shave some lemon zest into your water glass along with an ounce of fresh-squeezed lemon juice, suggests Glassman. Lemon peel contains pectin, a soluble fiber that has been shown to help with weight loss. The lemon boost also turns your beverage into an antioxidant power drink.

Helpful Bonus Tips

Those nine simple guidelines on the Eat Sheet are all you need for smarter, cleaner eating habits. Here are some optional things to do that you may find helpful.

ADD HERBS, SPICES, AND FLAVOR ENHANCERS TO EVERY MEAL.

You don't have to do this, but it really makes a difference. Herbs and spices perk up the flavor and add extra nutritional value, including antioxidants and antimicrobials for no (or very few) calories or milligrams of sodium. Even the *aroma* of spices can help you eat 5 to 10 percent less per meal, according to a recent study in the journal *Flavour*. "People may unconsciously take smaller bites to regulate the amount of flavor they experience," says study author Rene de Wijk, PhD, of Wageningen University in the Netherlands.

Your heart may benefit from a flavor boost, too: People who tossed 2 tablespoons of seasonings—such as black pepper, garlic powder, rosemary, paprika, cinnamon, and oregano—into a meal had 30 percent lower levels of triglycerides (a type of blood fat) afterward than those who didn't add a zing to their dishes. That's because certain spices may slow the digestion of fat, says study author Sheila G. West, PhD.

While they're not herbs and spices, hemp seeds, flaxseeds, chia seeds, and even crushed-up seaweed qualify as flavor enhancers. They add nutritional value, texture, and flavor. Just use a sprinkle as a topping. Here's a closer look at some important flavor enhancers.

Black Pepper

As mundane as black pepper may seem, it actually packs some metabolic punch. Piperine—the substance in black pepper that can irritate your nose—has been shown in animal studies to delay gastric emptying (so you feel fuller longer) and stimulate calorie burning, according to Dutch researchers.

TRY IT: On anything! Add it to stir-fries, roasted vegetables, meats, or even salads.

Cayenne and Chili Powder

The spicy capsaicin in cayenne revs up your body's internal furnace and keeps your insulin levels in check after a meal.

TRY IT: Sprinkle on a hard-boiled egg, salad, or homemade kale chips.

Chia Seeds

One tablespoon of chia seeds packs as much fiber as a bowl of oatmeal, plus bone-building calcium and heart-healthy omega-3s. They're also a good source of iron, which many women don't get enough of.

TRY IT: On cereal, salads, and soups, or use it to thicken pudding and stir-fries. Chia seeds absorb water, creating a gel-like consistency.

Cinnamon

This antioxidant-packed spice may help ward off the pounds by keeping your blood sugar in check, reducing your odds of storing fat while also curbing your appetite.

TRY IT: Stir into your coffee or on top of oatmeal or frozen yogurt.

Crushed Seaweed

Sure, it looks a little like fish food, but this stuff is nutritionally stacked. Seaweed is loaded with minerals, including calcium, and it's low in calories. And it's naturally salty, so you get that flavor with all of the minerals.

TRY IT: Sprinkle over a salad or to season vegetables or quinoa.

PICK YOUR PORTION

Taste Enhancers

When it comes to low- or no-cal herbs and spices, you can add as much zing as you want. Even so, we've included recommended portion sizes—enough to give you a nutritional benefit without overwhelming your taste buds. We've also listed portion sizes for more-caloric taste enhancers, such as honey, seeds, and dried fruit, which you should adhere to more strictly.

Coconut: 1 tablespoon

Dried fruits: 2 tablespoons

Dried seaweed: 1 tablespoon

Herbs (fresh, dry): to taste (~1 teaspoon)

Honey: 1 tablespoon

Nutritional yeast: ¼ cup

Seeds: 2 tablespoons

Spices (fresh, dry): to taste (~1 teaspoon)

Sun-dried peppers and roasted tomatoes: 1 tablespoon

Vanilla extract: 1 teaspoon

Vinegar (any type): 1 tablespoon

Ground Flaxseed

Flax is packed with fiber and ALA, a plant-based omega-3 fatty acid. Go for the ground-up kind: "When you grind flaxseeds, you get more benefit, because if you just eat them plain, they can go right through your system," says Glassman. Ground flaxseed is also a dynamite source of lignans, plant estrogens that may soothe monthly mood swings and help prevent overeating. And the fatty acids in flaxseed help hydrate your skin, according to German researchers.

TRY IT: Add to whole wheat pancakes or healthy muffins, or mix with whole wheat bread crumbs as a coating for chicken.

Hemp Seeds

First, let's clear the air: Hemp is *not* the same thing as marijuana. Unlike most plant sources of protein, these tiny seeds contain complete protein, which means that they're rich in all nine essential amino acids, not just a select few. (Just $1^1/_2$ tablespoons provides an incredible 5 grams of protein.)

TRY IT: On salads or roasted vegetables, stir into your morning oatmeal, yogurt, or soup, or blend into a smoothie.

Honey

Crave a shot of sweetness? Honey is your no-fail fix. "Yes, you're adding sugar, but you're getting sweetness with antibacterial properties," says Glassman. "Better to add a little bit of real honey than anything artificial."

TRY IT: Stir into yogurt or oatmeal or drizzle over natural peanut butter on a whole-grain cracker.

Oregano

Oregano—dried or fresh—is high in free radical–fighting antioxidants and has been shown to act as an antimicrobial.

TRY IT: With eggs, fish, or meat. Or spread a soft cheese, like goat cheese, on a cracker and sprinkle oregano on top.

Pumpkin Seeds

These power-packed seeds are loaded with iron and arginine, an amino acid that helps dilate your blood vessels, according to a study in the journal *Nutrition Research and Practice*. They're also a solid source of magnesium, a mineral few of us get enough of, and they contain cholesterol-taming phytosterols.

TRY IT: Sprinkle over a salad, in a trail mix, or grind into meal that can be added to flour for whole wheat pancakes or homemade bread.

Rosemary

The powerful oils in this herb stimulate circulation. Plus, rosemary is a proven memory booster.

TRY IT: On chicken or any other meat.

ASK THE LIFE STYLIST

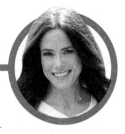

Keri Glassman, MS, RD, president of
Nutritious Life, in New York City

Q > I love cheese way too much to give it up. What are
the most weight-friendly varieties?

A < Quit cheese? No reason to! Eating cheese is an excellent
way to boost the calcium and protein in your diet, and
because it's filling, it can prevent overindulging later on. To
manage the calorie and fat downsides of cheese, watch your
portions. One ounce—that is, one deli slice, a 1-inch cube, or
2 tablespoons—has 75 to 100 calories. If you're looking for
naturally lower-calorie varieties, savor a little feta, Parmesan,
or goat cheese.

Q > There are so many Greek yogurts at the grocery
store. Are they all equally good for me?

A < It's no surprise that yogurt was one of the top foods
associated with weight loss in a 20-year study by the Harvard
School of Public Health: It's packed with protein and calcium,
and the Greek variety has even more—plus, its thick texture is
traditionally achieved by straining, which removes some of the
sugar and salt. But some companies use thickeners to create
that consistency, so check the ingredients panel for milk protein concentrate or cornstarch, two common thickeners. Watch
the flavored varieties, too, since they're often loaded with
added sugar. If you must eat them, stick to 6-ounce cups with
no more than 20 grams of sugar. Mix plain yogurt with some
berries and a little honey for a shot of fiber and antioxidants.

Turmeric

This bitter-tasting spice is derived from the dried root of a tropical plant. It's packed with curcumin, a compound thought to halt the growth of fat cells.

TRY IT: Mix into scrambled eggs or an omelet, or sprinkle into your cooking water when making quinoa.

CHOOSE YOUR OWN INDULGENCE FOOD WHEN YOU FEEL LIKE IT, AND ENJOY IT USING YOUR MINDFULNESS SKILLS.

If you follow the dietary guidelines in this chapter, you'll naturally displace some of the foods you used to live on—for example, if you're focusing on lean protein with every meal, you may no longer feel compelled to order a fatty burger for lunch. Or, as you work natural sources of fat into your daily diet, the unnatural sources—like doughnuts or potato chips—might fall off your radar. That said, there *is* room for indulgence, because your taste buds aren't going to automatically prefer kale chips to potato chips or fresh-picked blueberries over freshly baked blueberry pie. This means that having a portion-controlled treat can actually help you stay on track—especially in the beginning, when you're adjusting to this new way of approaching food.

Ideally, you'll indulge one to three times per week. You *can* choose to have a small indulgence every day, but before digging in, ask yourself if the cost of that treat is worth slowing your progress. If not, don't eat it—you'll just feel worse afterward. "Daily is a lot," says Glassman. "But if you're the type of person who feels deprived otherwise, go for it." If you know you're allowed to indulge, you avoid the deprivation mindset, which is often what drives us to eat foods that are in opposition to our goals. When the choice to indulge (or not) is yours—not just some rule you're being told you have to follow—you learn to listen to your body and have a treat only when you truly want one.

As you train your taste buds to enjoy—even crave—whole, nutritious foods simply by eating more of them, you may find that your indulgence of

PICK YOUR PORTION

Indulgences

When it's time to indulge, you can eat almost anything you desire—as long as you do so mindfully. If you pay attention while you eat—really savoring the experience and noticing your body's reactions—you may be surprised to find that a small portion really is enough to satisfy your yearnings. So what counts as a "small" portion? Here are suggested servings for commonly craved treats from Keri Glassman, MS, RD, president of Nutritious Life in New York City.

Chips: 10

Dark chocolate: $\frac{1}{2}$ ounce (about the size of half a Post-it note)

Cookie: 1 medium

French fries: $\frac{3}{4}$ ounce (10)

Gummy candies: 1 ounce (about 10 pieces)

Ice cream: $\frac{1}{2}$ cup

Nachos: 2 chips with $\frac{1}{2}$ ounce of cheese

choice changes naturally. During the first week of following this plan, you may want super-rich ice cream, but you may find that it tastes too sweet a few weeks later. Or if you're a salt lover, the tortilla chips you once craved may start to overwhelm your palate. "Sometimes, what was nonnegotiable [when you started] becomes negotiable 4 weeks in," says Lesley Lutes, PhD, an associate professor of psychology at East Carolina University. So right now, it may seem impossible to phase out your near-nightly bowl of Ben & Jerry's, but as you get back in touch with your body, you may find that you're willing to switch to fro-yo—or even cut back to ice cream only one night a week. But that's totally up to you—your indulgence is your indulgence.

If you find that your weight loss is stalling, this is the area where you have the most wiggle room: Tweaking your indulgences is an easy way to encourage the scale to start moving again. For example, if you hit a plateau, you might decide that you're willing to trade your Oreos for a lower-calorie cookie. Small changes can make a big difference—especially when you feel in control of those changes.

SNACK UP! EVERY SUNDAY EVENING, PREPARE SNACK PACKS FOR THE WEEK

Snacks keep hunger at bay so you don't run to the vending machine at work to stop for a doughnut. If you have them handy every day, you won't be tempted by calorie-dense packaged foods. Making your own at the beginning of the week helps you be proactive about mindful eating and gives you the goods for healthier snacking. Here are some quick ideas for creating a weekly arsenal of great snacks.

MAKE YOUR OWN FRUIT-AND-NUT TREAT. Cut up a large fresh apple and mix it with some chopped walnuts and a teaspoon or two of maple syrup. Or pack a plastic bag of apple slices and a small plastic container with a tablespoon or two of peanut or almond butter to tap the satiating power of nuts. A 2003 Brazilian study found that three apples a day can keep weight gain at bay—and can even help you lose.

CUT UP VEGETABLES. While making your dinners, cut up extra vegetables like carrots, celery, green beans, and yellow pepper to place in plastic bags to take to work the next day. Bring a small container of tangy hummus when veggies alone won't cut it for comfort food.

SINGLE-PORTIONS OF PACKAGED CHEESE. These make great on-the-go snacks. The protein and fat in, say, Sargento light string cheese snacks will keep you going until lunchtime.

GUILTLESS SNACK THAT TASTES LIKE DESSERT. Slice a cup of fresh strawberries and add 2 dollops of plain full-fat Greek yogurt for a sweet, fiber-rich combo.

SAVORY POPCORN. Toss some popcorn in a brown paper bag with cracked black pepper and parmesan cheese.

CANTALOUPE SQUARES. Cut up half a melon. Like most fruits, cantaloupe contains lots of water, so you fill up quickly—and get a great dose of beta-carotene—for not a lot of calories.

TUNA WITH MULTIGRAIN WHEAT THINS. Pack 2 ounces of tuna and a baggie of Wheat Thins for a high-protein snack that also contains energizing carbs and iron, which helps your muscles recover after a workout.

INSTANT OATMEAL. Keep packets of microwaveable instant oatmeal in your desk for a quick, filling snack. Studies have found that oatmeal is more filling than dry cereal with the same calories and fiber content.

KALE CHIPS. Skip the high-fat potato chips and pack these homemade chips. Bake some fresh kale leaves on a cookie sheet with a drizzle of olive oil. Top with sea salt. Kale is an awesome source of vitamins A, C, and K—plus calcium and fiber.

Meal Snapshots

The point of this plan isn't to dictate every bite you take—that'd be falling right into the overly rigid trap you're trying to avoid. But here are a few sample menus, based on the dietary guidelines in this book, to help you find your groove. Try them just as they are, or make a few tweaks based on your personal food preferences. Feel free to have fun and switch things up!

SAMPLE BREAKFAST #1

Toast a slice of sprouted-grain bread, and top it with a poached egg and a quarter of an avocado, cut into slices. Season with sea salt and cayenne pepper to taste.

The Breakdown

> MOOD FOOD: Avocado
>
> FAT: Avocado
>
> PROTEIN: Egg
>
> ANCIENT GRAIN: Sprouted-grain toast
>
> TASTE ENHANCERS: Sea salt and cayenne

SAMPLE BREAKFAST #2

Stir 2 tablespoons of dried cranberries, $\frac{1}{2}$ tablespoon of sunflower seeds, and $\frac{1}{2}$ tablespoon of chopped walnuts into 6 ounces of full-fat Greek yogurt. Add cinnamon to taste.

The Breakdown

> MOOD FOOD: **Walnuts**
>
> FAT: **Sunflower seeds**
>
> PROTEIN: **Greek yogurt**
>
> TASTE ENHANCERS: **Dried cranberries and cinnamon**

SAMPLE BREAKFAST #3

Add $\frac{1}{4}$ cup of nutritional yeast, 10 crushed almonds, 2 tablespoons of hemp seeds, and thyme (to taste) to $\frac{1}{2}$ cup of cooked steel-cut oats, prepared with water.

The Breakdown

> MOOD FOOD: **Steel-cut oats**
>
> FAT: **Almonds, hemp seeds**
>
> PROTEIN: **Hemp seeds**
>
> TASTE ENHANCERS: **Nutritional yeast, hemp seeds, thyme**

SAMPLE LUNCH #1

Combine $\frac{1}{2}$ cup of chopped tomatoes, a generous handful or two of fresh spinach, 2 artichoke hearts, 2 tablespoons of chopped red onion, and 4 to 6 ounces of roasted chicken. Sprinkle 2 tablespoons of flaxseed meal over the top, and dress with 3 parts balsamic vinegar to 1 part olive oil.

The Breakdown

> GREENS: Spinach, artichoke hearts
>
> MOOD FOOD: Spinach
>
> FAT: Flaxseed meal, olive oil
>
> PROTEIN: Chicken
>
> TASTE ENHANCERS: Flaxseed meal, balsamic vinegar

SAMPLE LUNCH #2

Add $1/2$ cup of sliced cucumber, 4 to 6 ounces of albacore tuna, and 2 tablespoons of hummus to $1/3$ cup of cooked quinoa. Toss it with 2 teaspoons of olive oil and 1 teaspoon of red wine vinegar, and sprinkle 1 tablespoon of fresh chopped parsley on top.

The Breakdown

> GREEN: Cucumber
>
> MOOD FOOD: Quinoa
>
> ANCIENT GRAIN: Quinoa
>
> FAT: Olive oil
>
> PROTEIN: Tuna, hummus
>
> TASTE ENHANCERS: Red wine vinegar, parsley

SAMPLE LUNCH #3

Tear off four leaves of romaine lettuce, and toss it with 4 ounces of firm, cold tofu (cut into $1/2$-inch chunks), $1/2$ cup of sliced red peppers, and $1/2$ tablespoon of thinly sliced scallion. Dress it with a blend of 1 teaspoon of peanut butter and 1 teaspoon of sesame oil. Sprinkle with 1 tablespoon of sesame seeds.

The Breakdown

> GREEN: Romaine lettuce
>
> MOOD FOOD: Red peppers
>
> FAT: Peanut butter, sesame oil
>
> PROTEIN: Firm tofu
>
> TASTE ENHANCER: Sesame seeds

SAMPLE DINNER #1

Bake $\frac{1}{2}$ sweet potato. Garnish $\frac{1}{2}$ of a baked sweet potato with 2 teaspoons of organic butter and $\frac{1}{4}$ teaspoon of dried oregano. Serve with 4 to 6 ounces of roasted coho freshwater salmon and a steamed artichoke.

The Breakdown

> GREEN: Artichoke
>
> MOOD FOODS: Salmon, sweet potato
>
> FAT: Organic butter
>
> PROTEIN: Salmon
>
> TASTE ENHANCER: Dried oregano

SAMPLE DINNER #2

Mix $\frac{1}{2}$ cup of cooked millet with $\frac{1}{2}$ cup of black beans. Top with $\frac{1}{4}$ medium avocado, cubed, and a dressing made from 1 tablespoon of Greek yogurt, finely chopped cilantro (to taste), 1 tablespoon of chunky fresh salsa, and 1 teaspoon of lime juice.

The Breakdown

> MOOD FOOD: Millet
>
> ANCIENT GRAIN: Millet

FAT: Avocado

PROTEIN: Black beans, Greek yogurt

TASTE ENHANCER: Cilantro

SAMPLE DINNER #3

In a foil pack, roast 4 to 6 ounces of cod with 2 teaspoons of olive oil, 2 table-spoons of sun-dried tomatoes, and rosemary, thyme, and lemon juice to taste. Serve with 12 medium stalks of steamed asparagus and $\frac{1}{2}$ cup of roasted red-skinned potatoes.

The Breakdown

GREEN: Asparagus

MOOD FOOD: Red-skinned potatoes, cod

FAT: Olive oil

PROTEIN: Cod

TASTE ENHANCERS: Sun-dried tomatoes, rosemary, thyme

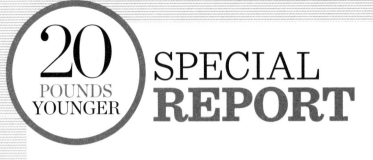

Your Probiotic Pantry

PROBIOTICS—THE LIVE MICROORGANISMS FOUND IN fermented foods such as kefir and kimchi—are one of the hottest, and most promising, topics in nutritional research. Your gut is teeming with trillions of bacteria that help you digest food as well as thwart intruders—and it turns out, you can give those friendly bacteria a boost by adding probiotics to your body. "We're only at the cusp of understand the potential of probiotics," says Gregor Reid, PhD, a microbiologist at the University of Western Ontario. Soon, Dr. Reid theorizes, probiotics may be used in prescription drugs to treat a range of conditions, from acne to depression.

There's another way these mighty microbes help your gut: In a recent study in the *Journal of Functional Foods,* people who ate probiotic-rich yogurt daily lost 3 to 4 percent of their body fat in 6 weeks. The shift in gut bacteria prompted by probiotics may favor fat burning over fat storage, explains study author Jaclyn Omar, of the University of Manitoba in Canada.

Some probiotics are much better than others. "The best, most natural forms of probiotics are fermented foods," says Lisa Ganjhu, DO, a gastroenterologist at New York University Langone Medical Center. Fortified foods, such as probiotic-enhanced dough, may deliver fewer of the good guys, since the manufacturing process can kill off many of the healthy live cultures. Besides yogurt, some common fermented foods include kefir (a fermented milk drink), sauerkraut (plus it counts as a veggie!), kombucha (fermented, sweetened black and/or green tea), kimchi (spicy pickled cabbage), miso soup, and fermented pickles. It's great if you can eat some fermented foods every day, but two or three times a week is a good place to start.

The amount and kind of live cultures per bite will vary, but words like raw, lacto-fermented, or unpasteurized on the packaging indicate that the bacteria haven't been killed off during the manufacturing process. Look for yogurt with the "live active cultures" seal; this indicates that it has not been heated after the fermentation process and contains at least 100 million cultures per gram (or 10 million cultures per gram for frozen yogurt).

Not sure where to start? Track down these proven sources of probiotics at your supermarket.

DANACTIVE YOGURT. Research suggests that this readily available yogurt can help ease some types of gastrointestinal distress. Eat it as a snack, or use it as the base for a delicious dip.

LIFEWAY FROZEN KEFIR. Kefir can improve digestion and restore beneficial bacteria after a round of antibiotics. Bonus: It has more protein and less sugar than yogurt, but with the same creamy texture and tangy taste. Try it in salad dressings or smoothies. Plain kefir is in the dairy aisle and can be consumed in all the same ways as yogurt, says Keri Glassman, MS, RD, president of Nutritious Life in New York City, but you'll find this dessert-ready kefir in the frozen foods aisle.

MAMA O'S PREMIUM KIMCHI. *Lactobacilli,* a type of good bacteria found in kimchi, can help prevent yeast infections. Kimchi is usually eaten as a side or garnish, says Glassman, who suggests pairing it with fish or vegetables.

REAL PICKLES ORGANIC SAUERKRAUT. A study published in the *British Journal of Nutrition* found that eating sauerkraut may help prevent cancer. Sauerkraut goes with more than hot dogs and Reuben sandwiches: You can eat it as a stand-alone side dish (it's a great substitute for slaw), on

NUT MILK = LIFE CHANGER!

I'm crazy about these awesome milk alternatives because I've learned that they taste wonderful and pack some serious nutritional perks. Nut milks are a great, nondairy source of calcium, since most are fortified with it. Just avoid the sweetened varieties. Here are some of my faves.

Almond Milk

Pour a glass of . . . Silk PureAlmond or Original Almond Milk

Although almond milk isn't packed with protein like the nuts themselves, it *is* a solid way to get a dose of calcium, as well as some vitamin B_{12} and riboflavin. Almond milk is an especially significant source of vitamin E. Plus, it's amazingly creamy and has a super-satisfying hint of sweetness. If you try another brand, make sure to choose one that doesn't contain carrageenan, an indigestible thickener often added to almond milk.

Cashew Milk

Pour a glass of . . . So Delicious Dairy Free Cashew Milk

top of lean chicken sausage and veggie or portobello burgers, or added to stir-fries (*after* cooking, to avoid killing the good bacteria). "Sauerkraut adds a sour note," says nutritionist Dawn Jackson Blatner, RD. "Chefs call it a brightener—it makes your food's flavor pop."

If you aren't getting enough probiotics from your daily diet, a supplement can make up the difference. Most supplements contain *Lactobacillus* and *Bifidobacterium*, although you'll see some with more strains (sometimes called "mega probiotics"). These pumped-up versions aren't necessarily better, but some experts say it's a good idea to switch supplements every month or two.

Recommendations vary, but supplements with at least 20 billion live organisms per dose tend to be most effective, experts say. You can choose from among powders, pills, and liquid shots, and some probiotics are sold

Cashew milk is a solid source of vitamins B_{12}, D, and A; in fact, it often contains more D than cow's milk. Expect a nutty, earthy taste that pairs well with a whole grain cereal.

Coconut Milk

Pour a glass of . . . So Delicious Dairy Free Coconut Milk

Coconut isn't truly a nut—but its milk is often lumped in with the others, since it has similar nutritional properties, including doses of calcium and vitamin D. Bonus: Coconut milk contains fatty acids known to kill plaque-causing bacteria in our bodies.

Hemp Milk

Pour a glass of . . . Tempt Hemp Milk Unsweetened Original

Hemp is technically a seed, but like actual nuts, hemp milk contains a dose of healthy fats—specifically, heart-healthy omega-3s. Other perks: This milk alternative fights inflammation, clotting, and high cholesterol, she says.

chilled and must be kept that way to maintain their effectiveness. Here are a few winners in the supplement world.

ALIGN. It contains *Bifantis,* a patented strain of bacteria that helps maintain digestive balance.

FLORASTOR. A study found that this supplement alleviates antibiotic-related diarrhea and may help boost the immune system, making this a smart choice when traveling, says Dr. Reid.

REPHRESH PRO-B. This is the only probiotic clinically shown to balance yeast and bacteria daily.

BE WELL BY DR. FRANK LIPMAN—PROBIOTIC POWDER. Add a teaspoon to your smoothie to ease chronic indigestion.

CULTURELLE DIGESTIVE HEALTH PROBIOTIC CHEWABLES. These have been shown to boost general digestive health.

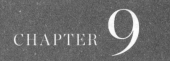

CHAPTER 9

Moves for a Strong and Sexy Body/Lift to Get a Lean Physique That Defies Gravity

> Weight training is the only way to *boost your metabolism* permanently. The more muscle you have, the more calories you burn 24-7.
>
> –HOLLY PERKINS, CSCS

OVER THE PAST YEAR, I STARTED TO NOTICE THAT MY Instagram feed was overflowing with images of superfit women, each photo emblazoned with a phrase such as, "Strong is the new skinny!" or "Cut the crap, ladies—lift!" Clearly, the idea of strength training has caught on in a big way. Still, many women are wary of lifting anything heavier than a hair dryer for fear of turning into an NFL linebacker. In fact, a recent university survey found that only a paltry one-third of people who do strength training are women.

Well, I'm hoping to change that. Strength training is a critical piece of the 20 Pounds Younger program because exercising your body with weights provides major health and antiaging benefits that you simply can't get as efficiently any other way. Every pound of muscle you add to your frame increases the number of calories you burn, even at rest, because muscle is more metabolically active than fat is, which means it requires more energy to sustain. With more muscle, you burn extra calories—even in your sleep!

"Strength is an often-overlooked component of physical health," says Alexander Koch, PhD, an associate professor of exercise science at Lenoir-Rhyne University. "Lifting weights is excellent for bone density, joint mobility, and body composition." And by body composition, he means that you'll look leaner and firmer—displaying the kind of sculpted muscle tone you've always dreamed of having. But let's stick with the health benefits of lifting weights for a second. We'll get back to aesthetics soon enough.

Weight-bearing exercise tugs on your skeleton, which stimulates your bones to lay down more bone cells, making your infrastructure stronger. The Health Professionals Follow-Up Study, an 18-year-long study of 32,000 men that was published in the *Archives of Internal Medicine*, also suggests that strength training is one of the best ways to control blood sugar and reduce your risk of type 2 diabetes. The analysis found that men who weight trained for at least 150 minutes per week had a 34 percent lower risk of type 2 diabetes than men who never hit the weights. The researchers say that resistance training improves the sensitivity of insulin receptors, which allows muscle cells to absorb glucose more easily, getting it out of your bloodstream quicker. Even though the study only monitored men, researchers say the results would be similar in women because muscle physiology is similar across genders.

The benefits don't end there. Resistance training can whip your psyche into shape, too: "Physical strength begets mental strength," says Jill Coleman, cofounder of the fat-loss company Metabolic Effect, based in Winston-Salem, North Carolina. "Finishing a tough weight-training session makes you feel like you can take on the world." And it can build confidence and an all-important sense of self-approval. In a 2006 study, McMaster University researchers found that women who did a strength training routine for 12 weeks experienced significant improvements in body image—concerning both how they felt about others checking them out and how satisfied they were with their own appearances.

If you are new to weight training or feel intimidated by gyms, the Life Stylists and other experts have your back: They'll break it down for you step-by-step, so you'll quickly gain the confidence to make resistance exercises part of your lifestyle for life. But first, let's bust some muscle myths to further convince you that the 20 Pounds Younger Fitness Plan is going to be your secret to a hot bod.

4 Myths of Strength Training

MYTH #1: *Lifting Weights Will Turn You into the Incredible Bulk*

No way. "The fear that you'll suddenly grow large amounts of muscle from lifting weights is akin to worrying that you'll be involuntarily drafted by the WNBA if you shoot a few hoops at the Y," says Dr. Koch. "Most of us don't have the genetic potential to develop really large muscles," adds Wayne Westcott, PhD, a professor of exercise science at Quincy College. And women are missing something else critical to building big-time muscle: testosterone. While you have some of the so-called "male hormone," you just don't have enough of this key muscle builder coursing through your body to inflate your biceps and lats. Westcott conducted one of the largest-ever studies comparing men's and women's muscle-building potential and found

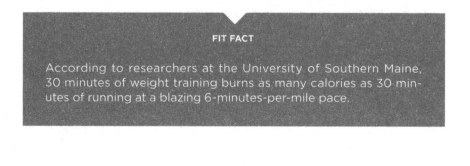

FIT FACT

According to researchers at the University of Southern Maine, 30 minutes of weight training burns as many calories as 30 minutes of running at a blazing 6-minutes-per-mile pace.

that after doing an identical weight-lifting routine for 10 weeks, the women in the experiment gained an average of 2.6 pounds of muscle, while men packed on 4.6. "The average age was about 50, so these people had lost a lot of muscle during the aging process," notes Dr. Westcott. "An average 20- or 25-year-old women wouldn't add that much muscle, because she hasn't lost any yet." Bottom line: No matter what your age, adding lean muscle to your frame won't bulk you up, but it will trim you down.

MYTH #2: *Muscle Can Turn into Fat*

Muscle and fat are two totally different types of tissue, so even if you slack off, that hard-earned muscle won't morph into fat. What it will do through lack of use is atrophy. If you lose muscle, you burn fewer calories, and if your food intake remains the same, the excess calories can be stored as fat. That's why maintaining muscle as you get older is so critical: Muscle is a significant calorie-burning engine that runs all day, every day.

MYTH #3: *Lifting Will Make You Gain Weight*

This is not so much a myth as a misunderstood truth. "Leaner" and "lighter" are not interchangeable terms, which means that the scale may not tip much (or may even tip in the wrong direction) when you start hitting the weights, says Chad Landers, owner of Push Private Fitness in Toluca Lake, California. Make no mistake: The physical results can still be dramatic. The more muscle you gain, the smaller and more compact you may become, so your pants may start to feel looser. "People get on the scale and say, 'I only lost 1 pound!'" says Dr. Westcott. "But I say, no, you made a 7-pound change—you gained 3 pounds of lean weight, and you lost 4 pounds of fat."

And that's *without* monitoring their diets. Pay a little attention to what you put into your body, and you'll only amplify your losses. In Dr. Westcott's research, people who cut back to about 1,500 calories while increasing their protein intake nearly doubled their fat loss. "This is not a low-calorie diet—it's fairly modest restriction," he says. "And you're still going to gain muscle."

MYTH #4: *Cardio Burns More Fat*

Walk into any gym and chances are, you'll find a herd of women gliding gazelle-like on the cardio equipment. Why do women flock to the treadmills and elliptical machines and forego the weights? With cardio, you perspire, so you're getting instant affirmation that you're making progress. But most of the weight you lose is water weight, Dr. Westcott says. I have to admit that I was once one of those cardio junkies. An aerobic workout session made me feel thinner, simply because I felt like I had done a lot of work. But here's what's so insidious about cardio training: with all that "sweat equity," I gave myself permission to overindulge as a workout reward.

That's the dirty little secret in the exercise world—cardio can actually make a girl fat. In a 2012 study in *Obesity Research and Clinical Practice*, males who jumped rope experienced no change in appetite. But females? You guessed it—their urge to eat shot up after the exercise session. One potential factor: Aerobic exercise may boost your body's output of ghrelin, one of the primary hunger hormones, and this hormonal effect seems to be exaggerated in women, say University of Wyoming researchers. But there's another factor at play, which I've noticed in myself. After aerobic exercise, the adrenaline rush creates a feeling of elation that drives us to splurge on a high-calorie snack as a reward. In a study published in the *Journal of Sports Medicine and Physical Fitness*, researchers found that people consumed up to three times more calories than they'd burned during an earlier workout. Why? The afterglow of a good workout may make us less mindful about what we put into our mouths, while also encouraging us to be less

---

FIT FACT

You are 61 percent more likely to skip a workout next week if you skip one this week.

active for the rest of the day. In a 2011 study, women burned 70 fewer calories during the day after doing a hard workout compared to days when they didn't hit the gym.

Afterburn: How Muscle Keeps You Lean for Life

Once you hit your thirties, your muscle begins disappearing at a rate of about 5 pounds per decade—and that amount doubles after you hit menopause. "That's like going from an eight-cylinder engine to a four-cylinder engine," says Dr. Westcott. "You don't burn as much energy, you gain fat that much faster, and you don't look as good because you're soft instead of firm."

Doctors have a term for what's going on. It's called *sarcopenia*. There's actually a sarcopenia laboratory that studies this phenomenon at the Jean Mayer USDA Human Nutrition Research Center on Aging at Tufts University. Researchers there found that sarcopenia starts in both men and women around age 30. You won't notice it happening because it's a very slow process where fat gradually infiltrates muscle tissue. Also, as you age, your body becomes less adept at synthesizing the protein you eat to sustain your muscle. This is how you can be fat even if you happen to be thin; you've no doubt heard the term "skinny-fat," which means you may not look big in clothes, but you have little muscle mass or tone when your clothes come off. A study in the *American Journal of Clinical Nutrition* found that for every pound of muscle a woman loses, she will typically gain a pound of fat. How? Well, if you don't hold on to your skeletal muscle as you get older, your body requires fewer and fewer calories to do all of those automatic life functions like breathe, pump blood, and check out hot guys. When your basal metabolic rate (BMR) declines, you'll put on weight even if you don't increase your food consumption. And here's the real bummer: You don't have to live a sedentary lifestyle for this to happen. It can occur even if you are aerobically active but are doing little to keep your muscles from shrinking.

INSTANT AGE ERASER

Daily Bum Firmer

Get on your hands and knees and bend your lower right leg toward your thigh. Keeping your knees bent, lift your right heel toward the ceiling. Hold this position for a few seconds, then lower to the starting position. Do 12 reps, then switch to your left leg and repeat. This move works 55 and 79 percent more of your hamstring and glute muscles, respectively, than squats alone, according to the American Council on Exercise.

Fortunately, there's a remedy: weight-bearing exercise. Resistance exercise (aka strength training) gives a one-two punch to your flab, since it helps you blast fat *and* build muscle. The fastest way to do both is to choose exercises that work multiple muscles at once, use a weight that's heavy enough to make the last few reps a struggle, and keep your rest periods short (around a minute). You'll learn exactly how to do just that with the 20 Pounds Younger Fitness Plan in chapter 10. Meanwhile, there's more good news to convince you that weights are worth a try.

With strength training, there's also a pretty cool perk called the afterburn, where you continue torching calories at an elevated rate even after you're done lifting. By Dr. Westcott's estimates, you'll burn around 250 calories during a 30-minute circuit-style workout (where you move fairly quickly from exercise to exercise) and then another 75 or 80 in the first hour afterward. He even has a name for this: the hour of power.

Some studies even show that people incinerate an extra 100 calories a day for 3 days after strength training! "One workout could increase your calorie burn over a 4-day period by 630 calories," says Dr. Westcott. "You don't get that from aerobic exercise, where you burn almost all of the calories during the session." Why does lifting give you such a big metabolic boost? Simple: Strength training creates microtears in your muscles and it takes several days—and lots of energy—to repair the tissue. And when your body repairs that tissue, you build more muscle and become stronger.

Overcome Your Fear of Heavy Metal

Weight lifting is kind of like salsa dancing: If you haven't tried it, it can be pretty daunting. You may be afraid of embarrassing yourself by not using the equipment correctly. Many women are self-conscious about their bodies and want to avoid being compared (or comparing themselves) to fitter women in the gym. Let's just call it what it is—*gymtimidation*. A 2011 study in the journal *Obesity* found that women who've experienced "weight stigma"—those who've felt discriminated against because of their size— often report feeling uncomfortable going to the gym.

Is that you? If so, there are two ways to deal with it. The first is to work out in the privacy of your own home. It's easy to set up some home strength-training options with a few pieces of inexpensive equipment. We'll explain how in the next chapter and share some of the many benefits of doing your workouts in the convenience of your own home.

The second is to get over your anxiety about health clubs, gyms, and heavy metallic objects. It's a worthy goal since working out in a gym has many benefits, too. The greatest is the community and camaraderie it offers. A gym is a great place to meet friends who share a common interest and similar health and fitness goals. And, of course, all of the important gear is right there.

To trigger the gumption to go for it, remember that just about everybody who walks through the door of a gym suffers a little bit of performance anxiety and embarrassment about wearing tight-fitting clothing. Then use these other tricks to pump yourself up for pumping iron.

DRESS FOR EXERCISE SUCCESS!

Think about your last date: Did you wear a muumuu? A schlumpy pair of jeans? Doubt it. The clothing you wear has a big impact on how confident you feel, which means you shouldn't hide behind baggy clothes at the gym, either. Body-hugging clothes make it easier to see your muscles working, helping you keep your form in check.

If you're new to this whole exercise thing, we suggest splurging on stylish workout clothes in colors and styles you love. It's a science-supported shopping spree: Research shows that when you like what you're wearing, you actually perform better in physical activities.

And don't forget your girls: Finding the right sports bra is critical to working out comfortably. Your breasts can move as much as 8 inches—up and down, side-to-side, and forward and back—during exercise, which can be pretty painful. In fact, one study found that 17 percent of women who experienced exercise-induced breast pain skipped a workout, reduced their exercise duration or intensity, or switched their activities because their hooters were hurtin'. Luckily, with advances in fit, support, and coverage, there's now a sports bra that's ideal for every activity.

Low-Impact Activities

Such as . . . Pilates, yoga, and floor-based workouts

What to look for: "Straps that stretch or adjust will stay on your shoulders when you bend, and a clasp-free back nixes pinching," says LaJean Lawson, PhD, an Oregon State University adjunct professor who studies the biomechanics of women's breasts during exercise. If you're big-breasted—a D cup or larger—look for a bra that's underwire, to lift and shape your ta-tas, with a padded back to cushion your spine.

Medium-Impact Activities

Such as . . . cross-training, cycling, weight training, and boot-camp classes

What to look for: "You need to find the sweet spot between support and the freedom to move," says Dr. Lawson. Find a bra that's not too tight around your ribs and that conceals cleavage. A firm band around your ribs will help keep things anchored.

High-Impact Activities

Such as . . . running, kickboxing, and contact sports

What to look for: To protect against bouncing, sweating, and chafing, opt for molded or underwire cups, wide straps (padded, if you're top-heavy), and fabrics such as polyester or nylon (with a little spandex, to hug and support).

CONFIDENCE BOOSTER #1: *Recognize Your Own Strength*

It's very unlikely that you're the weakest link in the gym. "The muscles in your body are just like everyone else's," says psychologist Jean Kristeller, PhD. In fact, even if you're overweight, your leg muscles are probably pretty well developed, since the heavier you are, the harder they have to work. Dr. Kristeller recalls a client who wanted to use the weight machines at her gym but was afraid she'd feel self-conscious, since she assumed she'd only be able to lift a small amount of weight. To her surprise, she found that the level she was using for leg exercises was much higher than what some of the much younger, thinner individuals could use. Lesson learned: Your body may surprise you if you give it the opportunity!

CONFIDENCE BOOSTER #2: *Don't Stress over Intensity*

A successful workout doesn't have to be training-for-the-Olympics intense. "People make the mistake of thinking of exercise as only vigorous activity," says Dr. Kristeller. "Strive to exercise at a moderate intensity, 'somewhat hard,' to obtain optimal health benefits," she says. The "talk test" can help you find this sweet spot: You should be able to speak a full sentence during exercise, but you shouldn't be able to carry on a conversation. Remember, your goal is to help your body—which requires being sensitive to its abilities, limitations, and needs. As your fitness improves, the intensity will come naturally.

CONFIDENCE BOOSTER #3: *Take a Group Fitness Class*

Walking into a body-weight boot camp class may sound like the last thing you'd want to do if you feel embarrassed in the gym, but you may be pleasantly surprised: New exercisers often flock to classes, since having an instructor close by can make them feel more comfortable, says Wayne Miller, PhD, who has studied exercise attitudes among overweight people. Consider calling ahead to find out if the class you're interested in is appropriate for beginners.

CONFIDENCE BOOSTER #4: *Breathe, Baby!*

Yoga's downward-facing dog pose and weight lifting's dumbbell bent-over row may seem worlds apart, but they share one common aspect: mindfulness. You can't do either well without self-awareness and focus, and it all starts with proper breathing. In weight training, it is important to inhale for 2 seconds during the load phase of an exercise (as you lower or prepare to lift). This stabilizes your core and increases the amount of oxygen in your bloodstream, boosting your aerobic capacity so you'll be able to work out harder, longer, and more effectively, says Andrew Braun, owner of Advanced Movement Studio in Appleton, Wisconsin. Exhale for 4 seconds during the exertion (lifting) phase. Whatever you do, don't hold your breath, which can spike your blood pressure and lead to dizziness.

CONFIDENCE BOOSTER #5: *Silence Your Inner Critic*

You may not be aware of it, but defeatist or negative self-talk—like thinking you have the biggest thighs in the health club—can prevent you from getting a great workout, says Chris Carr, PhD, a sport and performance psychologist at St. Vincent Sports Performance in Indianapolis, Indiana. Don't try to clear your head or avoid thinking, though—just watch your thoughts. "Once they tune into it, many women are stunned by how often they put themselves down with negative self-talk," says Dr. Carr. "Over time, critical thoughts may erode your motivation from the inside out." Mind gone off the rails? Simply breathe deeply, refocus, or trying reciting a mantra (see Confidence Booster #6).

CONFIDENCE BOOSTER #6: *Give Yourself a Pep Talk*

Before you walk into the gym and then again before every exercise, repeat a mantra—a word or phrase to help psych yourself up—that reflects the purpose of your workout. International fitness expert Brett Hoebel suggests thinking about a mantra like a hashtag: #strongbodystrongmind, #bestshapeofmylife, #fitfromwithin. If you're aiming to reduce anxiety and stress, try #justbreathe as your mantra. Want to feel strong? Go with #mindovermuscle. Mentally repeat your mantra throughout your workout—especially during the really tough parts, or when you catch your mind wandering. This really works.

CONFIDENCE BOOSTER #7: *Shut Out the World, Turn Up the Tunes*

Slipping in your earbuds during a workout might seem like an odd way to increase your focus—after all, plenty of us use music to mentally check out—but research shows that listening to certain types of tunes can actually help you keep your mind squarely on what you're doing. A study in the journal *The Sport Psychologist* found that tennis players reacted more quickly on the court when they listed to songs with an emotionally charged message (think "Eye of the Tiger" from *Rocky III*). "Songs with strong lyrical affirmations can give you a significant physical and mental boost when the going gets tough," says study author Costas Karageorghis, PhD.

Create a playlist of songs with lyrics or themes that speak to your intention for this workout—and crank up the volume when you feel you're starting to flag. If your intention is to "go faster," add Eminem's "'Till I Collapse," Kanye West's "Stronger," and Florence and the Machine's "Dog Days Are Over" to your list. Starting a fat-burning fire with interval training? Try "Burn" by Ellie Goulding. Looking to boost your mood? Crank up "I Gotta Feeling" by the Black Eyed Peas, "Beautiful Day" by U2, and "I Love It" by Icona Pop. "Choose as many songs as you need for your playlist to be effective and feed your intention," says Hoebel.

INSTANT AGE ERASER

Beat Fatigue with Music

Listening to music for about an hour a day can help reduce fatigue and may help your cells grow and repair themselves, keeping your insides spry, says biochemist Miguel-Angel Mayoral-Chávez, MD, PhD. Just make sure the beats are, well, upbeat, whether the music is Gaga or Mozart.

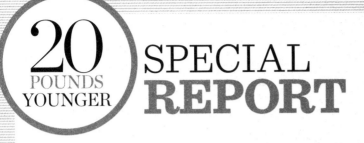
BLAST EVIL CELLULITE

DIMPLES ON YOUR CHEEKS ARE CUTE. But dimples on your butt cheeks—not so much.

Sadly, cellulite spares few women. By some estimates, 98 percent of us develop these stubborn lumps and bumps in unfortunate places like our tummies, thighs, and backsides.

"Cellulite is a neglected scientific topic—or better, a 'nontopic' for medical scientists," says Enzo Emanuele, MD, PhD, who wrote a paper summarizing cellulite treatments. "Cellulite was initially considered to be just localized accumulation of water and protein," Dr. Emanuele says. However, recent research has revealed that it's more like an internal traffic jam, "a complex structural alteration, due to reduced local bloodflow," he says.

In areas of your body where bloodflow is lacking—for example, your butt, if you sit for a large part of the day—there's also a shortage of oxygen, which can trigger inflammation and fibrosis, or internal scarring. When your skin starts puckering, the surrounding muscles may shrink from inactivity. As you lose your muscle tone, "you can start to see more of that saggy, cellulite-y skin," says Life Stylist Lauren Roxburgh, a personal trainer and expert in foam rolling. And if that's not discouraging enough, the physiology of cellulite is very similar to that of stretch marks, which means the two often coexist, according to a study review in the *Journal of the American Academy of Dermatology.*

But there's hope, and it may come in the form of a simple exercise tool: the foam roller. A foam roller is an inexpensive length of, typically, closed cell foam that's 6 to 9 inches in diameter and anywhere from a foot to 4 feet long. You guide your body over the roller back and forth, essentially giving yourself a deep tissue massage. Foam-rolling therapy is technically called self-myofascial release, and it works by alleviating adhesions or "knots" in soft tissue to restore elasticity and muscle motion.

"Foam rolling gives you more circulation, more oxygenated blood," says Roxburgh. "It's getting rid of congestion in the body." And it's one way exercise can help smooth out the cellulite. Buy a foam roller (at about $20, they are a lot cheaper than a masseuse!) and try these moves.

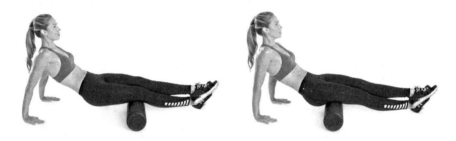

BACK-OF-THIGH ROLL

WHAT IT DOES: Breaks down and smooths tight, thick, and congested areas of the upper legs

Sit on the floor with your legs outstretched, then lift your butt and place the roller against the back of your upper thighs, just above your knees. Place your hands on the floor behind you for support, with your fingertips facing your backside. Put your weight on your hands, pressing into your palms, to lift your body up off the floor. Gradually push your body up and down so it moves over the roller under the backs of your thighs. Repeat 10 times.

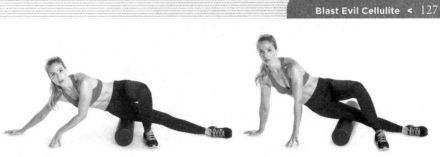

THE HIP ROLL

WHAT IT DOES: Narrows your hips by reducing fluid retention and smoothing out thickness in the connective tissue

Lie on your right side, and position the roller under your right hip, keeping your right leg extended on the floor. Bend your left knee, placing your left foot on the floor in front of you for support and leverage. Lift your torso, straightening your right arm, while keeping your hand planted on the mat for balance. Guide your body up and down the roller, along your outer thigh and hip. Repeat 10 times, and then switch sides.

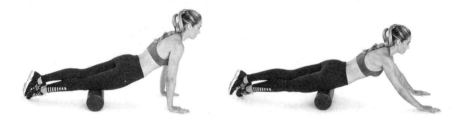

THE FRONT-OF-THIGH ROLL

WHAT IT DOES: Reduces bulkiness in your thighs by increasing circulation and aiding lymphatic drainage

Get down on all fours, then place the roller under your right thigh, just above your right knee. Bend your knees slightly (to lengthen your thigh muscles), and use your arms and core to gradually move the roller up your thigh and toward your hip, keeping your abs tight to avoid straining your lower back. Repeat 10 times, then switch sides.

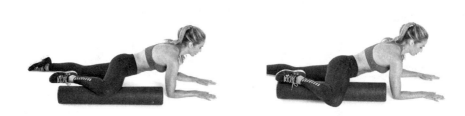

THE BENT-KNEE INNER-THIGH ROLL

WHAT IT DOES: Breaks down tissue density in the inner thighs and improves circulation to the area

Get into a pushup position. Place the roller between your legs against your right inner thigh, just above your knee. Bend your right knee, bringing your heel toward your butt, and bend your left leg, placing your knee on the mat. Roll up to your groin and back down again. Repeat 10 times, then switch sides.

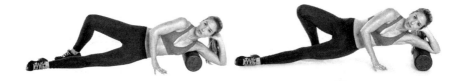

THE SLEEK ARMS ROLL

WHAT IT DOES: Helps reduce upper-arm jiggle and increases tone in your triceps by stimulating lymph nodes in your armpits to flush out built-up toxins

Lie on your right side with the roller under your right armpit so that it is positioned perpendicular to your upper arm. Push yourself so the back of your arm moves the roller toward your elbow and then back up into your armpit. Repeat 10 times, then switch to the other arm.

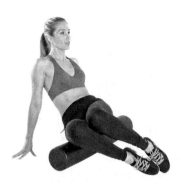
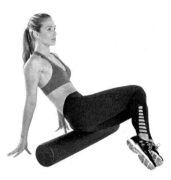

THE CAN-CAN TUSH ROLL

WHAT IT DOES: Reduces tissue thickness in your buttocks

Sit on top of the roller. Place your heels on the floor, and plant your palms on the floor behind you for balance, fingers facing away. Drop your knees down toward the right, then roll your hips and knees to the left. Continue rocking back and forth for 8 to 10 reps total.

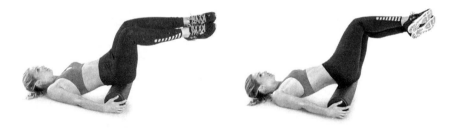

THE HIGH-TUSH ROLL

WHAT IT DOES: Reduces tissue thickness in your upper buttocks and helps stimulate lymphatic drainage (since you're upside down)

Lie flat on your back on the floor, and place the roller under your hips. Lift your feet off the ground and bend your knees until your weight is on the spot just above your tailbone. Place your hands on each end of the roller. Twist your knees, pelvis, and hips to one side, without moving your upper body, and then twist to the other side. Repeat 10 times.

THE BUTTERFLY ROLL

WHAT IT DOES: Stimulates lymphatic drainage—that is, it helps flush out clogged-up toxins in your tush and thighs

Sit on the roller with the soles of your feet on the floor and your knees bent (place your fingers on the floor outside your thighs for stability). Then bring the soles of your feet together, allowing your legs to open into a butterfly pose. Keeping your fingertips in place at your sides, use your hips and thighs to slowly move the roller forward and backward under your butt and thighs. Repeat 10 times.

ASK THE LIFE STYLIST

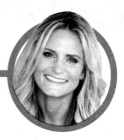

Lauren Roxburgh, foam-rolling expert, structural integration practitioner, and Pilates instructor

Q > Should foam rolling ever hurt?

A < You may feel discomfort—as in the hurt-so-good feeling of a deep-tissue massage. But you should never feel sharp pain (if you do, stop!), and the pain shouldn't linger into the following day (if it does, take a break from rolling for a few days). Start with light, quick motions and progress to slow, deep rolls. The whole point of rolling is to increase circulation, blood flow, range of motion, and flexibility, so take your time tuning in to each area. You want to allow your neuromuscular system to let go and relax.

Q > Are there any spots on my body I should avoid?

A < Yes! Avoid rolling over bony joints like your knees. Applying pressure could make you hyperextend your joints. It's good to get close to the attachment of the joints, but best not to go over them. Also, it's not recommended to roll back and forth on the lower back because it can create too much pressure or force on your discs and vertebrae. Lastly, you don't want to cause further inflammation by rolling each area for too long. Just a few minutes on each area will do the trick!

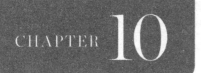

CHAPTER 10

6 Weeks to a Stronger, Younger You/Prepare to Feel More Powerful Than Ever (and Look Awesome Too)

THIS IS EXCITING. YOU'RE GOING TO BE STRONGER IN JUST 6 weeks. Your body is going to be firmer and tighter in places that used to jiggle. Best of all, you're going to love this exercise plan and, if you haven't done strength training before, you're going to wonder what took you so long to give it a try.

Here you'll find a strength-training program specifically designed for *20 Pounds Younger* by Life Stylist Holly Perkins, a certified strength and conditioning specialist based in Los Angeles. As a female trainer, Perkins knows what we're all up against when we hit the weights. And she's spent her career figuring out the most effective ways to train women's bodies, including her own, which—believe me—is an inspiration.

"Women's bodies are anatomically different than men's bodies—we're bottom-heavy, they're top-heavy," she says. "So the way we train our muscles needs to be different."

Perkins designed the 20 Pounds Younger Fitness Plan specifically for what most women want: well-toned, firm muscles that enhance their natural assets. Yes, it's a body reshaping plan, but it's more than that, too: It's a functional workout—one that's built to make everyday movements (for example, carrying groceries) easier by building strength in the areas you need it most. "In order to be muscularly balanced, you need to do more pulling exercises than pushing exercises," says Perkins. "That's why this workout has a two-to-one ratio of back to chest exercises." That kind of workout helps reduce your risk of shoulder injury and improves your posture by strengthening your posterior (back-of-body) chain of muscles, which is one of the best ways to look leaner and younger. Remember: Slouching ages you visually and breaks down your spinal health. Anything you can do to stand tall will improve your energy and even the way you look in clothes.

The Fitness Plan

You will do three workouts per week: two strength-training workouts and a "metabolic" workout designed to really crank up the fat and calorie burning. It's simple, built for beginners, but can be adapted as your fitness advances (or if you're not new to weight training but are just looking for a more effective program). Best of all, it's designed to get you back to your busy life in 30 minutes.

HOW IT WORKS

> **Warm up.** Do the warmup exercises each time you work out. Wrap up your workout with the cooldown exercises.

> **Work out.** Alternate between the three different workouts—Strength Workouts A and B, and the Metabolic Workout, performing each once a week.

> **Rest.** Allow for 1 day of rest between each workout. So if you do Workout A on Monday, for example, you might do Workout B on Wednesday or Thursday and the Metabolic Workout on Friday or Saturday. The rest

days are very important; your body needs an adequate amount of recovery time to repair the microtears that occur in your muscles during resistance training. This repair process burns calories even though you are resting, and it's how your body lays down firm, lean muscle. You are encouraged to play sports or go for a walk or easy run during rest days (you'll see this referred to as Fun Fitness below), as long as you aren't pushing your body too hard. Rest means not stressing your muscles so they have time to repair.

> **Progress.** After about 2 weeks, increase the amount of resistance or weight you are using for the exercises. By the end of 6 weeks, you'll have bumped up the weight of your dumbbells twice—and if you choose to continue this exercise routine, you'll increase the amount of weight you're lifting again at the conclusion of the 6 weeks. Want to keep challenging yourself? Continue increasing the weight you use until you reach your goals for your body.

SAMPLE WEEKLY WORKOUT SCHEDULE

Monday	Workout A
Tuesday	Rest or Fun Fitness
Wednesday	Workout B
Thursday	Rest or Fun Fitness
Friday	Metabolic Workout
Saturday	Rest or Fun Fitness
Sunday	Walk or Run

WHAT YOU NEED

> Dumbbells, in a range of sizes. At the very least, you should have two sets: one light (5 to 10 pounds) and one heavier (12 to 15 pounds or more). Any gym will have these. If you intend to work out at home, snag a used set of dumbbells at a garage sale for cheap. Once you're hooked, you'll likely be eager to add pairs of 8- and 20-pound dumbbells for more versatility.

> An exercise bench is optional but useful.

> An area that's about 6 by 10 feet where you can exercise without hitting anything (if you are planning to exercise at home).

KNOW THE LINGO

Warmup: just what it sounds like—you warm up your muscles.

Cooldown: easy, active recovery designed to bring down your heart rate after a workout.

Repetitions or reps: the number of times you perform a complete exercise.

Sets: the number of times you perform the required repetitions.

Circuit: a round of three or more exercises performed one after another with little to no rest in between.

ASK THE LIFE STYLIST

Holly Perkins, CSCS, author of
Lift to Get Lean

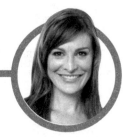

Q > I've been told it's impossible to spot-train. True?

A < That's a big fat myth. Here's why: The areas women tend to want to spot-train—triceps, bra fat, muffin top—are places with higher body fat. Dieting alone won't specifically target these spots, but exercise can. I make it happen all the time. The science backs this up: In a study in the *American Journal of Physiology,* researchers found that fat cell breakdown was higher in adipose tissue near a muscle being exercised, compared to fat tissue adjacent to a resting muscle. This suggests that exercise is, in fact, capable of spot-reducing the areas being challenged.

Q > How do I know if I'm working out hard enough?

A < When it comes to training with weights, there's an easy way to know whether the weights you are using are heavy enough to give you an efficient and effective workout. I call it the two-rep rule, and it goes like this: The weight you're using is heavy enough if you have to struggle to complete the last two repetitions of your set. In other words, your form should start to break down because you are so fatigued by the time you get to your last two reps. That's a good sign that you're pushing yourself hard enough. If, at the end of your set, you feel as if you could have knocked out more reps, you aren't working hard enough. Add more weight. It's only by continuing to challenge your muscles that you'll reap all the benefits of weight training.

WARMUP EXERCISES

You might be tempted to skip over this part to get to the main workout, especially if you are pressed for time. Please don't. Exercising with cold, tight muscles is a good way to get injured. It's like trying to tie your shoes with frozen shoelaces. Besides, research has shown that dynamic stretches (or what you know as grade-school calisthenics) prime the mind-muscle communication grid, which improves performance and boosts fat burning. Jumping jacks, running in place, arm circles, and squat thrusts are all good, classic ways to get your blood pumping, but on the next page is a five-move drill that'll ensure you warm up every part of yourself. And it's quick: Do one round of each exercise without resting between moves, a workout style known as a circuit.

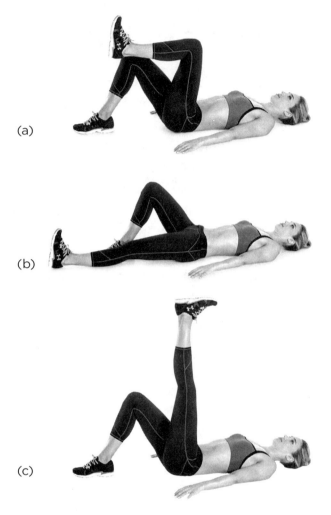

(a)

(b)

(c)

1. LYING RUNNER'S CYCLE

STARTING POSITION: Lie flat on your back with your knees bent and your feet flat on the floor (not shown).

THE MOVE: Draw your left knee toward your chest (a), pause briefly, and then extend your left leg straight out, so it rests on the floor (b). Now swing from your hip, raising your left leg straight up toward the ceiling (c). That's one cycle. Complete 10 cycles with each leg. You can do all 10 with one leg before moving to the other leg, or you can alternate legs.

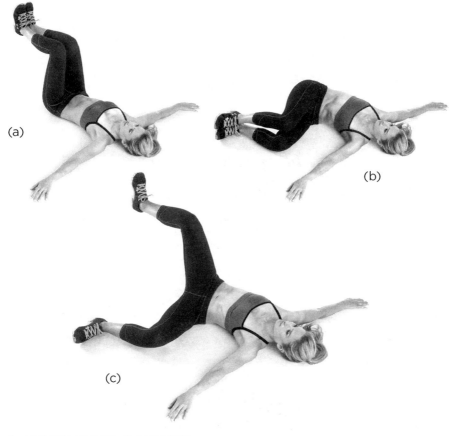

(a)

(b)

(c)

2. WINDSHIELD WIPER

STARTING POSITION: Lie flat on your back with your knees bent and your feet flat on the floor. Extend your arms out to your sides so your arms and hands rest on the floor and your palms are facing down. Lift your feet so that your shins are parallel with the floor (a).

THE MOVE: Keeping your knees together, drop them to your left side, pivoting from your hips and keeping your shoulders in contact with the floor (b). Next, leave your left leg on the floor, and spread your right leg to the right until you feel a stretch in your inner thigh (c). Lift your left knee to meet your right and drop both knees to your right side. Leave your right leg on the floor and spread your left leg to the left. Raise your right knee to meet your left. That's 1 rep. Continue alternating from side to side until you've performed 20.

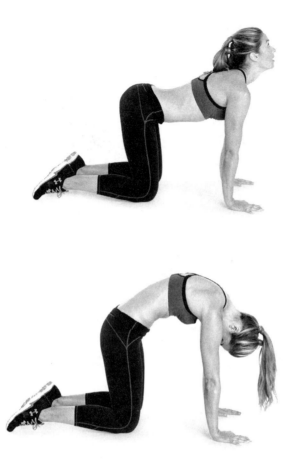

3. COW AND CAT

STARTING POSITION: Get down on all fours with your toes pointed behind you. Your hands should be directly under your shoulders, your thighs perpendicular to the floor, and your knees hip-width apart. Keep your head in line with your back and look between your hands.

THE MOVE: Keep your arms straight as you inhale, drop your belly, lift your head to look forward, and roll your shoulders back (Cow). Exhale, press your weight into your palms, round your upper back, drop your head to look down, and drop your tailbone down (Cat). That's 1 rep. Do 10.

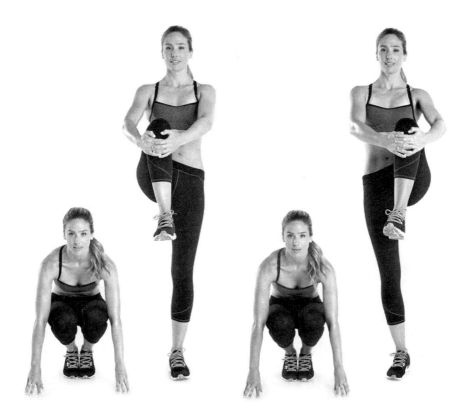

4. CROUCH TO STANDING KNEE PULL

STARTING POSITION: Start in a crouched position, balancing upright on your toes, with your knees to your chest and your fingers on the floor in front of you.

THE MOVE: Stand up and lift your right knee up to your chest, grasping it with both hands just below your kneecap. Release your leg, and return to the starting position. Stand up and draw your left knee to your chest. Release your leg, and return to the starting position. That's 1 rep. Complete 10.

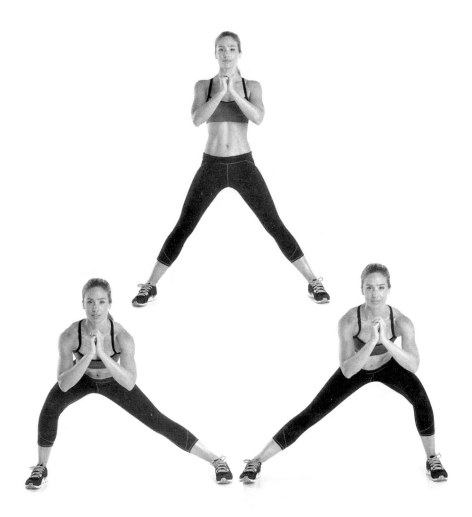

5. WIDE LEG SIDE SIT (LATERAL LUNGE)

STARTING POSITION: Stand in a wide stance (feet about twice shoulder-width apart) with your toes pointed forward. Clasp your hands in front of your chest.

THE MOVE: Shift your weight over to your right leg as you push your hips backward and lower your body by dropping your hips and bending your knees. Without raising yourself back up to a standing position, reverse the movement to the left. That's 1 rep. Do 20.

STRENGTH WORKOUT A

There are eight exercises in this workout. Perform one exercise after another, circuit-style at a comfortable pace, with no rest between exercises or circuits. Complete three full circuits. For each exercise, perform 15 reps for the first set, increase the weight and do 12 reps for the second set, and increase the weight again and do 10 reps for the third and final set, as indicated in the chart below. Note that you will increase reps of the All Fours Crunch, but no weight will be used.

"The muscle starts firing on your first set," says Perkins. "By the third set, you're physiologically more prepared to lift a heavier weight. Your muscle has really kicked into gear." Aim to increase your weight for each set every 2 weeks. For example, if you initially performed your 15-rep set with 10-pound dumbbells, you might progress to 12-pound dumbbells after 2 weeks.

Time: 30 minutes

CIRCUIT	REPS OF EACH EXERCISE	SUGGESTED STARTING WEIGHT (WEEK 1)
Circuit 1	15	10 pounds
Circuit 2	12	12 pounds
Circuit 3	10	15 pounds

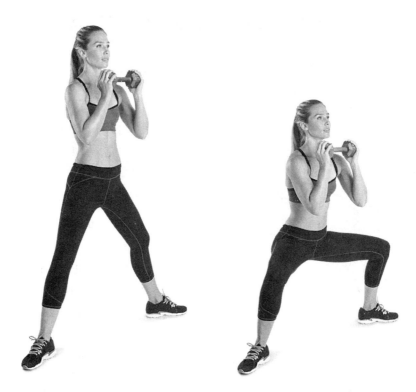

1. DUMBBELL SUMO SQUAT

Targets: quads and calves

STARTING POSITION: Stand with your feet about twice shoulder-width apart, toes turned out slightly. Keep your weight on your heels for the entire movement. Grasp a single dumbbell with both hands, wrapping your fingers around each end of the weight. Bend your elbows so you're holding the weight at your shoulders, keeping your upper body tall and erect. Don't flare your elbows out to the side. Keep them pointed toward the floor.

THE MOVE: Push your hips back and bend at your knees to lower your body until your thighs are parallel to the floor. Pause, then slowly return to the starting position.

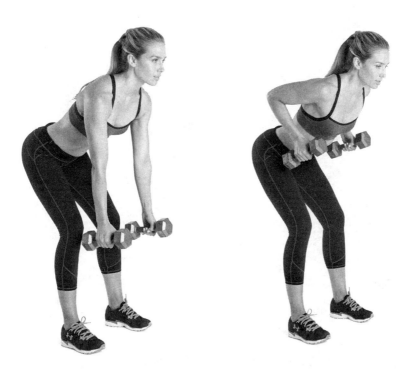

2. BENT-OVER DUMBBELL ROW

Target: upper back

STARTING POSITION: Stand with your feet shoulder-width apart. Hold a dumbbell in each hand, arms down at your sides. Bend at your hips and knees, and lean forward so your chest is almost parallel to the floor. Allow the weights to hang at arm's length straight down from your shoulders, palms facing each other.

THE MOVE: Bend your elbows, pulling the dumbbells to the sides of your torso while keeping your elbows close to your body. Pause, then slowly lower the dumbbells.

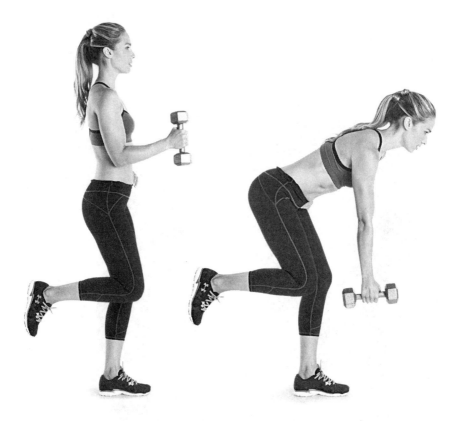

3. STEP-FORWARD TOUCH DOWN

Targets: glutes and hamstrings

STARTING POSITION: Stand with your feet together. Grasp a light-weight dumbbell in your right hand and bend your elbow at a 90-degree angle. Bend your left knee slightly, and pick your right foot up off the ground, bending your right knee so your lower leg is parallel to the ground.

THE MOVE: Lean your torso forward and extend your right arm, lowering the weight toward the floor. (You don't have to touch the floor, but do so if you can without compromising your form.) Return to the starting position. Complete all reps on one side, and repeat on the opposite side.

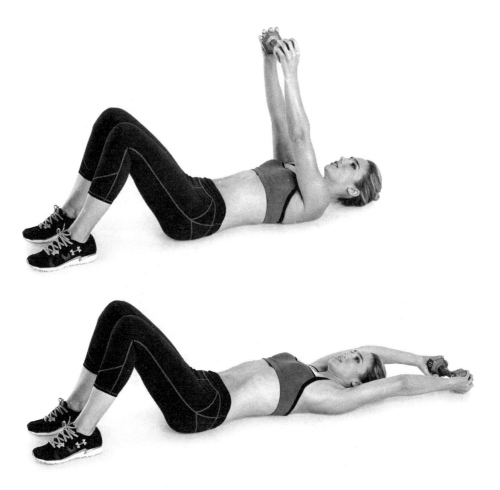

4. LYING STRAIGHT-ARM DUMBBELL PULLOVER

Targets: lats and triceps

STARTING POSITION: Lie flat on your back with your knees bent and your feet on the floor. Grasp both ends of a dumbbell, and straighten your arms overhead so the weight is directly over your chest.

THE MOVE: Keeping your arms straight, slowly lower the weight in an arc behind your head until you feel a stretch in your chest. Return to the starting position.

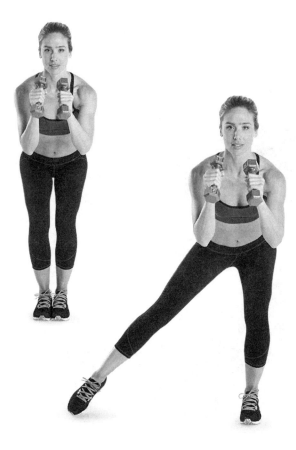

5. ISOMETRIC NARROW SQUAT WITH SINGLE-LEG SIDE TAP

Targets: quads and calves

STARTING POSITION: Stand with your feet together and your knees nearly touching. Hold a dumbbell in each hand with your palms facing each other, and bend your elbows to bring the weights to your chest.

THE MOVE: Push your hips back and bend your knees into a squat. Keeping your left leg bent, swing your right leg out, touch your toe to the floor, pause, and return to the starting position. Complete all reps on one side, and repeat on the opposite side.

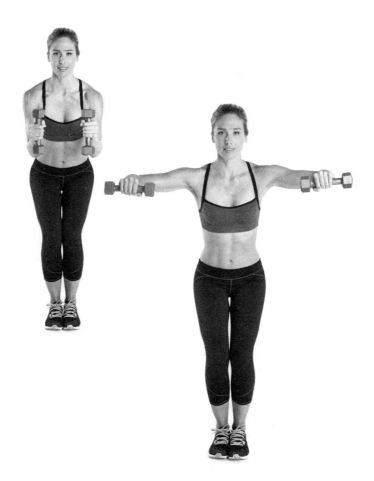

6. BENT-ARM DUMBBELL SIDE RAISE

Target: shoulders

STARTING POSITION: Stand with your feet together. Hold a dumb-bell in each hand and bend your elbows at 90-degree angles, palms facing each other. Bend slightly forward at the waist and also bend your knees.

THE MOVE: While maintaining the bend in your elbows, swing your arms up and out to your sides from your shoulders until they're paral-lel to the floor, palms facing down. Pause and return to the starting position.

7. ALTERNATING DUMBBELL BICEPS CURL

Target: biceps

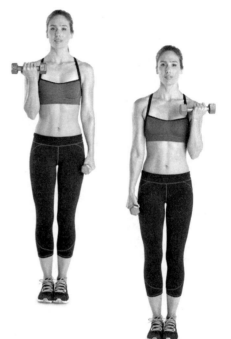

STARTING POSITION: Stand with your feet together and hold a dumbbell in each hand, arms straight down by your sides and palms facing each other.

THE MOVE: Bend your right elbow, curling the weight to your right shoulder as you rotate the dumbbell so your palm faces toward you. Return to the starting position, then bend your left elbow, curling the weight to your left shoulder. Continue alternating sides.

8. ALL FOURS CRUNCH

Target: abs

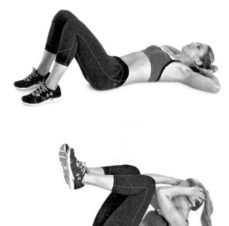

STARTING POSITION: Lie on your back with your knees bent and your feet on the floor. Place your hands behind your head with your elbows out to your sides.

THE MOVE: Lift your head and shoulders off the floor, pull your elbows forward, and draw your knees to your chest, touching your thighs to your elbows. Return to the starting position.

STRENGTH WORKOUT B

There are eight exercises in this workout. Perform one exercise after another, circuit-style, without resting in between exercises. Continue until you have completed three full circuits, taking 1 minute of rest between each circuit. Perform 15 reps of each exercise for each circuit, using a weight that makes your last 2 reps difficult. You may end up using the same weight during all three circuits—and that's okay, as long as the final couple of reps challenge you. Every 2 weeks, try to increase the pounds used for each lift so that, again, your last two reps are always difficult to complete. Note that some of the exercises in this workout are performed without weights.

CIRCUIT	REPS PER EXERCISE	RECOMMENDED STARTING WEIGHT (WEEK 1)
Circuit 1	15	10 pounds
Circuit 2	15	12 pounds
Circuit 3	15	15 pounds

Time: 30 minutes

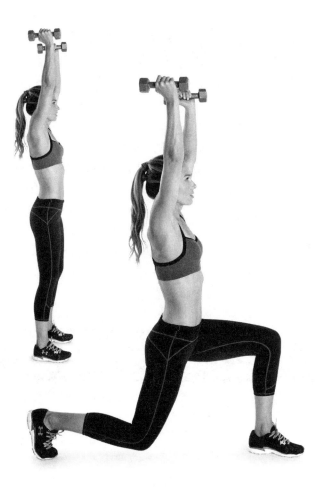

1. DUMBBELL REVERSE LUNGE

Targets: quads and calves

STARTING POSITION: Stand with your feet hip-width apart. Hold a pair of dumbbells above your head at arm's length, palms facing each other. Stand tall with your shoulders pulled back.

THE MOVE: Step backward with your right leg, and slowly lower your body until your front knee is bent at 90 degrees, keeping your lower leg nearly perpendicular to the floor. Pause, then push yourself back to the starting position as quickly as possible. Complete all reps on one side, then repeat on the opposite side.

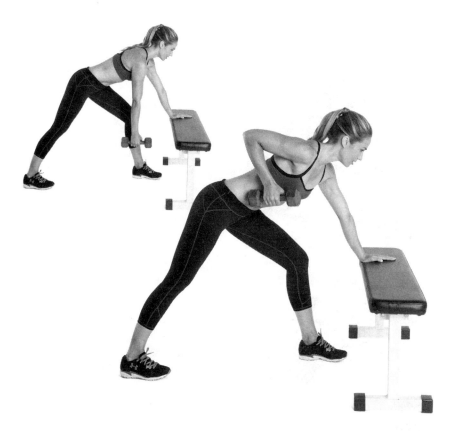

2. SUPPORTED BENT-OVER DUMBBELL ROW

Target: upper back

STARTING POSITION: Stand in front of an exercise bench or chair with your feet spread about 18 inches apart and your left foot a large step forward of your right. Lean forward from your hips, and place your left hand flat on the bench or seat of the chair. Grasp a dumbbell in your right hand, and let your right arm hang straight down toward the ground, palm facing inward.

THE MOVE: Bend your elbow, pulling the dumbbell up to the side of your torso while keeping your elbow close to your body. Pause, then slowly lower the dumbbell. Complete all reps on one side, then repeat on the opposite side.

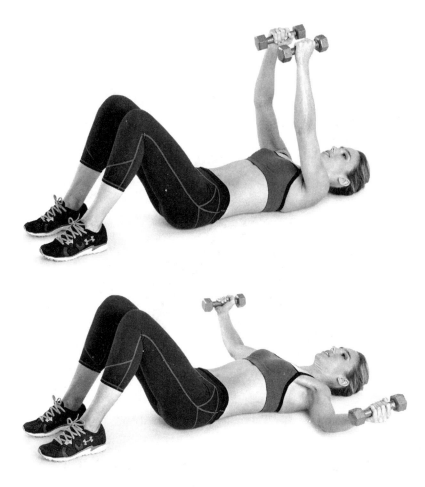

3. LYING DUMBBELL FLY

Target: chest

STARTING POSITION: Grab a pair of dumbbells and lie flat on your back on an exercise bench or the floor. Keep your knees bent and your feet flat on the floor. Hold the dumbbells over your chest with your elbows slightly bent and your palms facing each other.

THE MOVE: Without changing the bend of your elbows, slowly lower the dumbbells out to your sides and slightly back until your upper arms are parallel to (or touching) the floor. Pause, then return to the starting position.

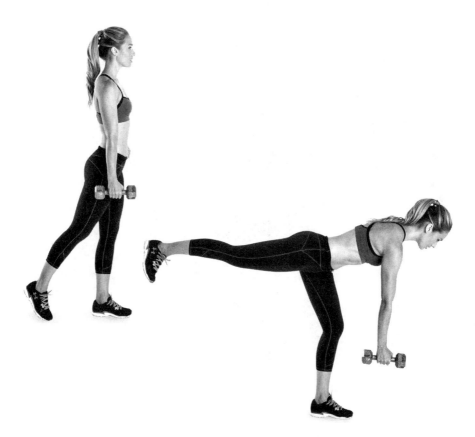

4. SINGLE-LEG DUMBBELL DEADLIFT

Targets: glutes and hamstrings

STARTING POSITION: Stand with your feet together, and hold a dumbbell in your right hand, hanging straight at your side.

THE MOVE: Lift your right foot off the floor so you're balancing on your left leg. Slightly bend your left knee, bend at your hips, and lower your torso until it's almost parallel to the floor and allow your right leg to rise behind you. Keep your right arm extended down and your right leg parallel to the floor. Pause, then raise your torso back to the starting position. Complete all reps on one side, then repeat on the opposite side.

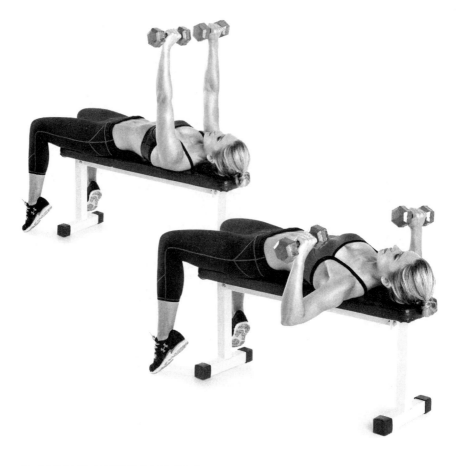

5. LYING CHEST PRESS WITH DUMBBELLS

Target: chest

STARTING POSITION: Grab a pair of dumbbells and lie flat on your back on an exercise bench or the floor. Keep your knees bent and feet touching the floor. Extend your arms straight up toward the ceiling, directly over your shoulders, with your palms facing your feet.

THE MOVE: Without bending your wrists, bend your elbows to lower the dumbbells to the sides of your chest or to the point where your elbows hit the floor, if you're on the floor. Pause, then press the weights back up to the starting position. Straighten your arms completely at the top of each rep.

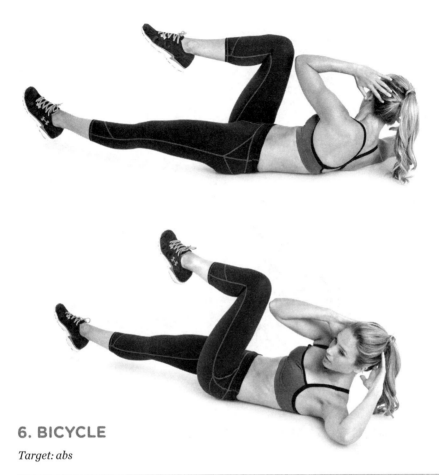

6. BICYCLE

Target: abs

STARTING POSITION: Lie on your back on the floor with your hips and knees bent at 90 degrees so that your lower legs are parallel to the floor. Place your fingers on the sides of your head, elbows out to your sides. Lift your head and shoulders off the floor.

THE MOVE: Use your abs to twist your upper body to the right as you pull your right knee in toward your left elbow, simultaneously straightening your left leg. Then twist to the other side and switch your legs so that your left knee reaches toward your right elbow and your right leg is straight. This is 1 rep. Continue alternating sides.

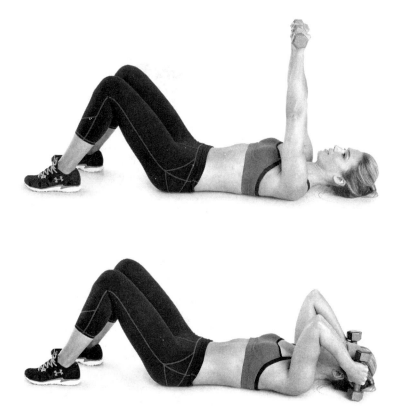

7. ROTATING DUMBBELL FRENCH PRESS

Target: triceps

STARTING POSITION: Lie flat on your back, with your knees bent and feet flat on the floor. Hold a dumbbell in each hand and extend your arms straight overhead, so the dumbbells are above your chest, palms facing toward your feet.

THE MOVE: Keeping your upper arms perpendicular to the floor, bend your elbows to lower the dumbbells toward your ears while rotating your hands so your palms are facing each other. Pause, then return to the starting position, rotating your palms to face toward your feet again.

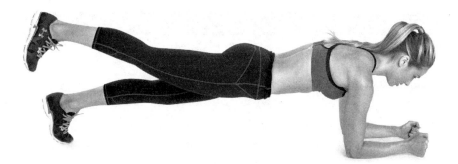

8. ALTERNATING SINGLE-LEG ELBOW PLANK

Target: core

STARTING POSITION: Start to get into a pushup position, but bend your elbows and rest your weight on your forearms, instead of on your hands. Your elbows should be directly under your shoulders. Move your feet out wider than your shoulders. Keep your body in a straight line from shoulders to ankles through the entire exercise. Squeeze your glutes and don't allow your hips to sag.

THE MOVE: Raise your right foot a few inches off the floor. Brace your core by contracting your abs. Hold the leg elevated for 3 seconds, lower it, and repeat with the opposite leg. That's 1 rep.

METABOLIC (FAT-BLASTER) WORKOUT

This no-weight routine torches calories while building cardiovascular fitness, strength, and power—all in about 20 minutes. Perform each exercise for 30 seconds, rest for 10 seconds, and move on to the next exercise. Complete the prescribed number of circuits, with 1 minute of rest between each circuit.

Weeks 1 and 2	2 circuits
Weeks 3 and 4	3 circuits
Weeks 5 and 6	4 circuits

Time: 18 minutes

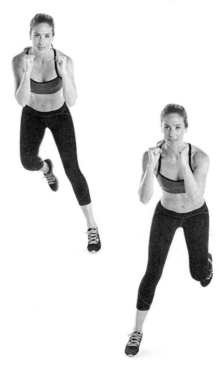

1. LATERAL SIDE JUMP

STARTING POSITION: Stand on your left foot, with your right knee bent and your foot raised off the ground in front of you. Bend your elbows, and hold your hands at your chest for balance.

THE MOVE: Jump to your right and land on your right foot with your left knee bent and your left foot in the air. Keep jumping back and forth, alternating landing legs.

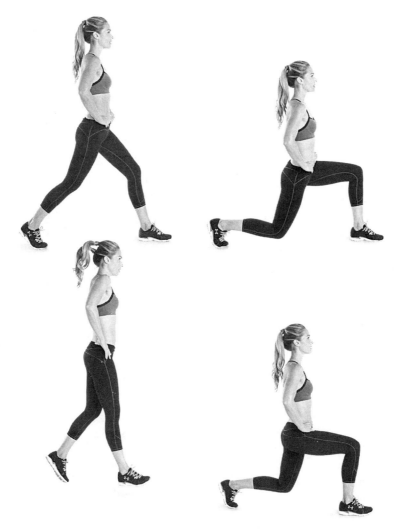

2. SPLIT-SQUAT JUMP

STARTING POSITION: Stand with a staggered stance, your left foot in front of your right. Place your arms on your hips.

THE MOVE: Bend your left knee, forming as close to a 90-degree angle as possible, and lower your right knee toward the ground. Jump and alternate your legs, so you land in the same position, but with your right foot in front and bent at almost 90 degrees. Continue jumping and switching legs.

3. BODY-WEIGHT SQUAT

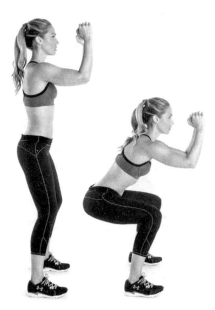

STARTING POSITION: Stand with your feet slightly wider than hip-width apart, and bend your elbows so your forearms are parallel to your chest, with your hands in front of your face.

THE MOVE: Bend your knees slightly and then initiate the move by pushing your hips back as if to close a door behind you with your butt. Lower your buttocks toward the floor until your thighs are parallel to the floor. Pause, then quickly return to the starting position and repeat.

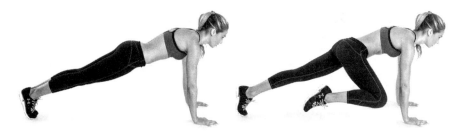

4. MOUNTAIN CLIMBER

STARTING POSITION: Assume a pushup position, with your arms totally straight and your hands under your shoulders. Keep your body in a straight line from your shoulders to your ankles, without letting your hips sag.

THE MOVE: Lift your right foot off the floor and slowly raise your knee as close to your chest as you can. Touch the floor with your right foot, then return to the starting position. Repeat with your left leg. Continue alternating sides.

5. JUMPING JACK

STARTING POSITION: Stand with your feet together and your arms at your sides.

THE MOVE: Simultaneously raise your arms out to your sides and over your head and jump your feet out so they are slightly wider than shoulder-width apart. Without pausing, quickly reverse the movement and repeat.

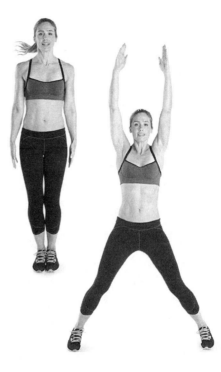

6. HIGH-KNEE JOG IN PLACE

STARTING POSITION: Stand tall with your elbows bent at 90-degree angles at your waist, palms facing down.

THE MOVE: Run in place, hopping from foot to foot and alternately lifting each knee as high as you can, trying to tap your hands with your knees. Your thighs should be as close to parallel to the floor as possible.

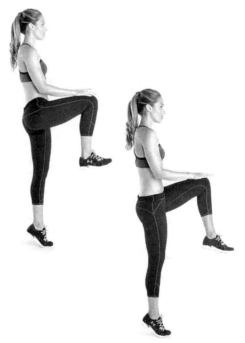

SCULPT YOUR ABS!

Add these belly-blasting moves to your routine at least twice per week.

Lying Anchored Leg Lowering

Starting Position: Lie flat on your back with your knees bent and your feet flat on the floor. Grasp a dumbbell in each hand and extend your arms straight above your chest, palms facing toward your feet. Press the ends of the dumbbells together, raise your legs, and bend your knees so your lower legs are parallel to the floor and form a 90-degree angle with your thighs.

The Move: Extend both legs straight up toward the ceiling, then lower your right straight leg toward the floor. Bring it back up, and lower your left leg. Raise your left leg. That's 1 rep. Continue alternating legs for 10 reps. Do 2 sets.

Lying Dumbbell to Knees

Starting Position: Lie flat on your back with your knees bent and your feet flat on the floor. Use your hands to grasp both ends of a dumbbell, and extend your arms straight up over your chest.

The Move: Swing your arms back over your head, dropping the weight toward the floor behind you. Activate your abs to lift your hips off the ground while bringing the dumbbell up over your head until it touches your knees. Reverse the movement, lowering your butt to the ground and bringing the weight from your knees to the floor behind your head. Complete 2 sets of 25 reps.

Down Dog into Plank

Starting Position: Start in Downward-Facing Dog (see Modified Pigeon on page 166).

The Move: Shift your weight forward and your hips downward, straightening your legs and arms so you're in pushup position. Your body should form a straight line from head to heels. Shift your hips up and back to return to Downward-Facing Dog. Do 2 sets of 20 reps.

COOLDOWN EXERCISES

An active recovery—that is, moving as a way to relax after your workout—can help your body bounce back faster. You have options when it comes to your cooldown: Head outside for a brisk 15-minute walk; crank up your music and dance like mad for the length of one song; or hit the treadmill, elliptical, or stationary bike for 8 to 10 minutes. Or simply perform these three exercises.

1. HALF SUN SALUTATION

Stand tall with your feet together, arms at your sides, and shoulders down. Inhale, and lift your arms straight up over your head. Exhale as you bend from your hips, and fold forward, touching your fingers to the floor if possible. Your back should remain flat throughout the movement. Inhale and pivot up from your hips. Keeping your knees slightly bent, place your hands on your thighs just above your knees, and look out in front of yourself. Exhale as you fold forward again, straightening your legs, rounding your back, and allowing your arms to hang down toward the floor. Hinge at your hips to return to standing, raising your arms overhead. Lower your arms to return to the starting position. Complete 5 reps.

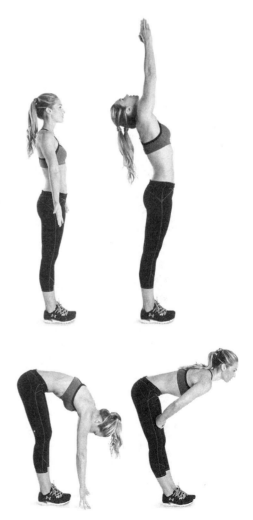

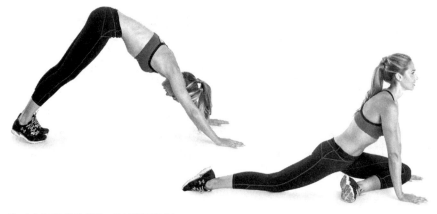

2. MODIFIED PIGEON

Start by getting into the Downward-Facing Dog pose, placing your hands flat on the floor and shoulder-width apart, your hips hinged so your butt is in the air, and your body raised up on the balls of your feet (see photo above, left). Now, bring your left knee in toward your chest. Place your left foot on the floor behind your right wrist and lower your hips, pivoting so your left knee rests on the floor and your calf is parallel to your chest. At the same time, drop your right knee to the floor and tuck your foot in toward your butt. Drop you chest toward the floor so it rests against your left calf. Hold for 30 seconds, then repeat on the opposite side.

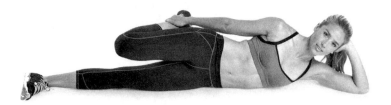

3. SIDE LYING QUAD STRETCH

Lie on your left side with your knees straight and your left arm extended above your head. Bend your left elbow to support your head with your hand. Bend your right leg, bringing your heel to your butt, and hold on to it with your right hand. Keep your thigh parallel to the ground and avoid lifting your knee up into the air. Hold for 20 seconds, then switch sides. Stretch each leg twice.

THE PERFECT HOME GYM

You don't need a squat rack or even a barbell. You can get a great strength-building workout using just a few simple tools—many of which can easily be stowed in a closet. Buy the highest quality equipment that you can afford, says Life Stylist Holly Perkins.

Stability Ball

These giant bouncy balls may look like they belong on a playground, but they're actually one of the most versatile pieces of exercise equipment out there. (They're essentially a less-stable version of an exercise bench.) For most women, a 55-centimeter ball is the right size, although taller gals should opt for a 65-centimeter ball. "Keep it blown up firm," says Perkins.

Resistance Bands

These rubber band–like cords come in a range of sizes and levels of resistance. Perkins's advice? Spring for three different stretchy bands: light, medium, and moderately heavy resistance. "Buy all of your bands from one company—don't mix and match brands," says Perkins. Why? One company may use green tubing for their lightest band, while another uses green for its heaviest band. "It just gets confusing," she says. Look for a set that comes with a door anchor, so you can hook your resistance band to the hinges, giving you more exercise options.

Dumbbells

Ideally, you'll have five sets of dumbbells: 5-, 8-, 10-, 12-, and 15-pounders. That way, you can select the exact weight you need for each exercise—and make sure you're practicing with proper form while still challenging your muscles.

(continued)

Exercise Mat

No matter what type of flooring you have, an exercise mat is a worthy investment. "You should have one even if you have carpet, which can make you slip and slide," says Perkins. Plus, giving yourself a little extra cushioning relieves pressure on your joints when you're doing exercises like planks. Keep in mind that an exercise mat isn't the same thing as a yoga mat (although you can invest in one of those, too). The material shouldn't stretch like yoga mats generally do, and it should be a little thicker.

Foam Roller

You can use this simple piece of equipment to massage worn-out muscles, or you can incorporate it into your actual workouts (see page 126 for details). Look for a solid, medium-density foam roller with a smooth surface.

BONUS EQUIPMENT: Exercise Bench

We get it: Exercise benches are ugly—and kind of expensive. That said, "if you have an exercise bench, you can do everything," says Perkins. In other words, this piece of equipment is what distinguishes a so-so home gym from a superb one. For about 50 bucks, you can get a basic bench—one that's long enough to rest your head and feet on while your knees are bent. If you opt for a pricier adjustable bench—one that can lie flat or have an upright back—make sure the gap between the two cushions is minimal. "If there's a big gap, it hits right around your tailbone and butt," says Perkins. That could leave your lower half unsupported—exactly what you *don't* want.

CHAPTER 11

Yoga, Your Way / Simple Poses for Mindfulness, Relaxation, and Body Toning

Yoga is not a religion. It is a science, science of well-being, *science of youthfulness,* **science of integrating body, mind, and soul.**

– AMIT RAY, *YOGA AND VIPASSANA: AN INTEGRATED LIFESTYLE*

DESPITE THE WILLOWY WOMEN YOU FIND IN MANY YOGA studios, most styles aren't sufficiently strenuous to help you lose a significant amount of weight, says Alan Kristal, DPH, MPH, a professor of epidemiology at the University of Washington, who has studied yoga and weight loss. But that doesn't mean yoga shouldn't be part of your 20 Pounds Younger routine.

Look beyond the physical part of the practice and you'll find valuable exercises in self-awareness, relaxation, and mindfulness—all of which can go a long way toward helping you reach your goal weight, says Judith Hanson Lasater, PhD, PT, and author, who has taught yoga for more than 40 years. "Yoga is about turning inward and paying attention: 'How's my posture? How is this pose stretching me? How's my breathing? Am I feeling tense?'" she says. This type of thinking eventually extends off the mat, helping you pay attention to internal cues like hunger or emotions that drive you to eat.

This may explain why yoga devotees are some of the slimmest people in the gym. In one study, Dr. Kristal found that middle-aged people who practiced yoga for as little as 30 minutes a week for 4 or more years gained less weight over a decade than nonpractitioners—and the difference in weight gain was as much as 18.5 pounds! So if it typically doesn't burn tons of fat, how does yoga keep you svelte? "It makes you less reactive to discomfort," he explains. "You take a pose to your personal edge—you don't push or hurt yourself, but you learn to be in a somewhat challenging position with equanimity." In other words, you realize you *can* stay put, even when your muscles are burning—and that may translate into greater tolerance for sensations such as stress or sadness that tempt you to eat a cheeseburger for breakfast.

Through Life Stylist Kathryn Budig, yoga teacher at YogaGlo.com and author of *The Women's Health Big Book of Yoga*, I've discovered that yoga can help me to feel more powerful and in control of my thoughts and body. One of Budig's mantras is, "You have to stop before you can start." This means that if you slow down, physically and mentally, you put yourself in a position to have a better workout and a better day.

How Yoga Changes Your Mind and Body

If you've ever taken a yoga class, you've probably experienced its seemingly paradoxical effects on your mood: You feel at once powerful and more Zen. Amazing, right? Well, you're not the only one who's noticed the incredible impact of yoga on mental health. In a recent *International Journal of Yoga* study, obese people who practiced poses for 1 hour a day, 5 days a week, experienced greater reductions in depression and anxiety than aerobic exercisers did after 6 months of exercise. And a new study published in the journal *BioPsychoSocial Medicine* found that 12 weeks of yoga training helped rein in women's anger, fatigue, and anxiety, while also relieving their medically unexplained health woes, such as headache, nausea, and lower back pain.

How can a physical activity have such a therapeutic effect? Simple: Done properly, certain yoga sequences induce a state that's the opposite of stress, both mentally and physically, says Budig. (The Sanskrit word *yoga* is the root source of the English word "yoke," meaning to connect.) Yoga is about connecting mind and body; no wonder it's one of the best things you can do to boost positive feelings about your whole self.

If you are not currently practicing yoga, you can reap many of the benefits without joining a studio. You can easily guide yourself through yoga sequences in your living room, at your own convenience. On the following pages, you'll find descriptions of basic yoga poses that will help you start forging this mind-body connection. The poses are a terrific way to work your way up to the strength-training program in the previous chapter, if need be, or to simply use once or twice a week as a regular element in your 20 Pounds Younger program. Here are two great routines from Budig's home practice book, *The Women's Health Big Book of Yoga*.

THE RELAXATION SEQUENCE

Do the following sequence of eight poses anytime you're feeling anxious or it's time to wind down for sleep at bedtime.

ALTERNATE NOSTRIL BREATHING

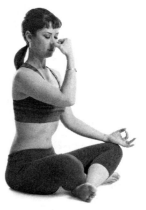

Tuck in the index and middle fingers on your right hand. Place your ring finger on your left nostril and your thumb on your right. Close off your right nostril and inhale normally through your left. Release your thumb and close your left with your ring finger and exhale evenly through your right. Inhale through your right again. After you inhale, close the right and exhale through the left. Continue for at least 1 minute or 5 breath cycles.

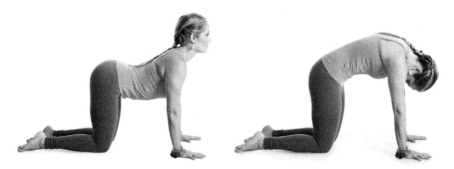

COW AND CAT

Start on all fours with your hips stacked over your knees and your shoulders stacked over your wrists. Keep your arms straight as you inhale, drop your belly, and roll your shoulders back (this is Cow). Exhale, press into your palms, round your upper back, and drop your tailbone down (this is Cat). Repeat this several times, performing Cow on the inhale and Cat on the exhale, to warm up your spine.

STANDING FORWARD FOLD WITH VARIATION

Stand with your feet hip-width apart. Exhale as you extend forward from your hips, keep your legs straight, and fold forward to the floor. Elongate your core, and keep your hips stacked over your heels. Interlace your fingers behind your back, and then drop your arms forward so they're parallel to the floor. Squeeze your arms as close together as possible and lengthen as you bend toward the ground.

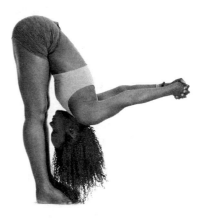

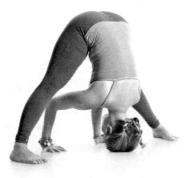

WIDE-LEG FORWARD FOLD

Start with your feet parallel and one leg-length apart. Put your hands on your hips and engage your quads. Keep rooting yourself in the outer edges of your feet as you hinge forward from your hips, moving your hands to touch the floor shoulder-width apart. Inhale as you extend your chest and straighten your arms. Exhale as you walk your hands as far back as they'll comfortably go, bending your elbows at 90-degree angles and placing the crown of your head on the floor (or as close to it as you can get). Keep your elbows over your wrists and your shoulders lifted.

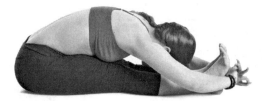

SEATED FORWARD FOLD

Sit on the floor with your legs together and extended straight out in front of you. Root into your hips and lift your chest. Keep your spine long and lean forward to grab the outer edges of your feet or, if you can't reach them, clasp your right wrist with your left hand. Inhale and extend your chest. Exhale and, without rounding your back, lengthen your torso over your legs. Relax your neck and shoulders. Press your thighs down and keep your feet flexed.

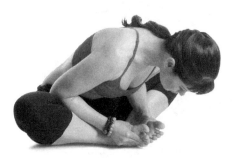

BOUND ANGLE

Sit on the floor and bend your knees, bringing the soles of your feet together, toes pointed forward and heels close to your pelvis. Grab hold of your feet and separate the soles like you're opening a book. Keep holding on to your feet as you fold forward, pulling your belly toward your feet and your head toward the floor. Avoid rounding your spine. Use your elbows to pin your legs down and help your knees come closer to the floor.

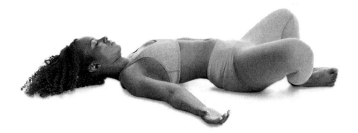

RECLINED BOUND ANGLE

Lie on your back with your knees bent and spread wide and the soles of your feet together. Bring your heels as close to your pelvis as you comfortably can. Lift your chest and draw your shoulder blades down your back to lengthen your neck. Stretch your arms wide out to your sides, with your palms facing up.

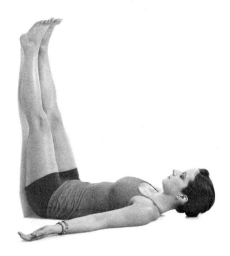

LEGS UP THE WALL

Sit on the floor next to a wall. Bend your knees and lie back on the floor. Pivot your torso and extend your legs up the wall so your hips and the entire length of the backs of your legs rest against the wall. (It's optional to use a strap to tie your feet together so your legs can relax even further.) Let your arms rest next to you, palms up.

THE CORE SEQUENCE

We all want a bikini-ready midsection, and let's face it: A strong core requires effort. Pretend you're a ninja as you move through this sequence and you'll get through it in no time—strong, calm, quiet, and slick! The goal here isn't to see how many reps you can pump out in a short amount of time. Take the time to breathe and make your movements thoughtful and precise.

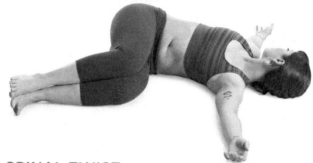

SIMPLE SPINAL TWIST

Lie on your back and hug both of your knees to your chest. Open your arms wide, palms up, keep your knees bent and together, and drop your legs to your right side. Push your left shoulder down as you elongate your lower back and turn your head slightly to the left. Return to the center and repeat on the opposite side.

FIT FACT

Regularly practicing yoga can produce favorable changes in your body composition. For example, yoga can shift your ratio of muscle to fat, even when your overall weight stays the same, according to a 2013 University of Arizona review of yoga research.

THE YOGA-PANT TRAP

You don't have to go to a yoga festival to see hordes of women in black stretch pants—just walk into any mall or supermarket. These days, women treat yoga pants like everyday streetwear. According to one survey, nearly a third of us think it's acceptable to wear yoga pants all the time. That may not be a good idea if you are trying to lose weight. "Wearing yoga pants allows you to eat a lot, whereas you'd be really uncomfortable if you wore more fitted things, such as jeans," warns Katie Rickel, PhD, a clinical psychologist and weight-loss expert who works at a weight-management facility in Durham, North Carolina. "You can lose perspective about when things are getting tight, because yoga pants are so forgiving."

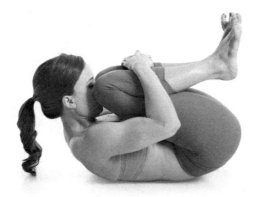

TINY LITTLE PACKAGE

Lie on your back and draw both knees to your chest. Grab your shins, pulling your legs tight to your chest, and draw your forehead or even nose toward your knees so that your head leaves the ground. Relax your shoulders.

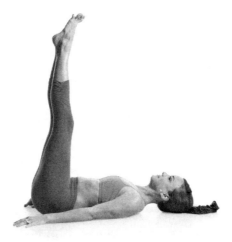

LOWER-BELLY LIFTS

Lie flat on your back with your legs straight up in the air. Rest your arms at your sides, palms down, and relax your shoulders. Exhale as you lift your hips a few inches off the ground. Inhale as you lower back down.

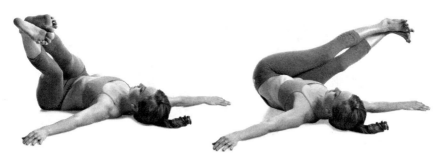

WINDSHIELD WIPER ABS

Lie flat on your back with your legs straight up in the air. Rest your arms straight out to your sides on the ground so that your palms are facing down and are in line with your shoulders. Exhale and keep your legs straight and together as you lower your legs toward one side, reaching your feet toward your hand. Inhale to come back up to center, and then switch sides. Cross your ankles for extra support to keep your legs straight, focus on squeezing your upper, inner thighs together to activate adductors.

6 TIPS TO MAXIMIZE MAT TIME

1. Dress appropriately.

You should wear comfortable clothes that are form-fitting but not restrictive. Avoid clothes with zippers, snaps, and pockets.

2. Find the right time for your practice.

If you work out in the morning, when your body temperature is lower, allow yourself a little extra warmup time. And if you work out late at night, beware: Since exercising raises your heart rate and temperature, you may have trouble falling asleep.

3. Be consistent.

If you hope to use yoga as a weight-loss tool, you need to limber up at least three times per week, according to a study review in the journal *Alternative Therapies in Health and Medicine.*

4. Keep breathing!

If you're holding a pose, you shouldn't be holding your breath. Establish a rhythm of inhaling and exhaling, before your practice: Inhale into your belly, then your ribs, and finally your chest, then as you exhale, reverse the order, breathing out through your chest, ribs, and lastly your belly.

5. Push yourself, but don't hurt yourself.

Move to a point of stretch but not strain. As long as you aren't in pain, you should try to hold the pose until your instructor says it's time to let go. A little muscle fatigue won't hurt you.

6. Don't compare yourself to others.

There *will* be some more advanced yogis in your group. Resist the urge to measure your back bend against theirs.

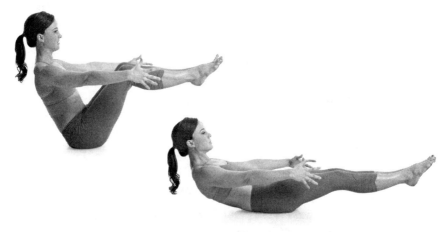

BOAT WITH BENT KNEES INTO HALF BOAT

Sit on the ground with your knees bent. Keeping your spine long, lean back just far enough so that your feet float off the ground. Keep your knees bent and legs pressed together as you lift your shins parallel to the floor. Extend your arms forward and parallel to the ground. Stay balanced on the tripod of your tailbone and sit bones, chest lifted and gaze forward. Hold for 5 breaths, and repeat 5 times.

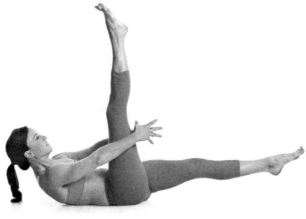

FINGERTIP ABS

Lie flat on your back with your legs straight up in the air. Keep your right leg up and lower your left leg until it hovers above the ground. As you exhale, curl your head and chest off the ground and extend your arms forward. Hold this position or, if possible, join your fingertips together in front of your right hamstring. Repeat with the opposite leg.

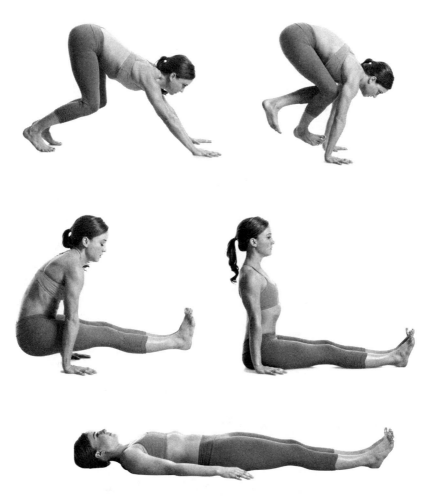

VINYASA AND JUMP-THROUGH TO LIE-DOWN

Start in Downward-Facing Dog (see Modified Pigeon on page 166). Step your feet together and look way past your hands, where your feet will eventually land. Keep your eyes on this spot as you come onto the balls of your feet. Bend your knees and hop up, pulling your thighs as close as you can to your torso, and flex your feet as they pass between your arms. Keep pressing your hands into the ground to pull more strength into your core. Let your heels land first, then your bottom. Lie flat on your back, with your legs extended straight out.

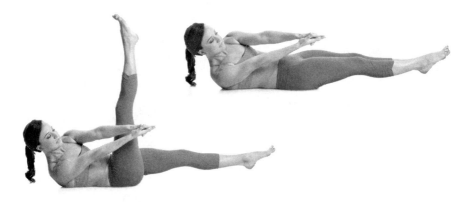

TWISTED LOWERING ABS

Lie flat on your back with your legs straight up in the air. Keep your right leg up and, keeping your left leg straight, lower it until it hovers above the ground. As you exhale, curl your head and chest off the ground and extend your arms to the outside of your right thigh, interlacing your fingers. Exhale as you hold your twist and lower your top leg to meet your bottom leg. Inhale as you lift your right leg back up to its original position. Switch legs and repeat.

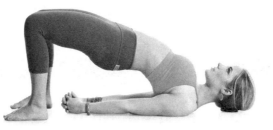

BRIDGE

Lie on your back with your knees bent and your feet flat on the floor, hip-width apart. Lift your hips off the floor enough to interlace your fingers beneath your lower back. Place your shoulders under your chest and press into your feet to lift your hips up as high as your knees. Keep a slight lift in your chin and allow your bottom to be soft. Your knees should stay in line with your hips as you rotate your inner upper thighs downward to broaden your lower back.

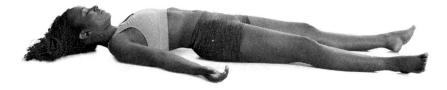

CORPSE (SAVASANA)

Lie on your back. Let your legs and arms flop open with your palms facing up. Lift your chest to snuggle your shoulder blades down your back. Release all tension in your body. Close your eyes (or even better, cover them with a cloth) and bring your breathing back to normal. Empty your mind. Take a rest.

ASK THE LIFE STYLIST

Kathryn Budig, yoga teacher
at YogaGlo.com and author of
The Women's Health Big Book of Yoga

Q > I have only 15 minutes to do yoga. Is it even worth bothering?

A < Any time on the mat is better than no time on the mat, especially if you're using yoga to combat stress. Even I sometimes find myself limited to short yoga sessions—often just 10 or 15 minutes—and I have learned that simply being disciplined about carving out time, however little, helps me stay committed to my daily practice. If you want to make sure your quickie workout is intense enough, try doing flow-style yoga, where you seamlessly transition from one move to the next, to help elevate your heart rate.

Q > Is it okay if I eat before yoga class?

A < Avoid eating for 2 hours beforehand. The primary concern is that you'll feel totally uncomfortable twisting and contorting into crazy postures if your belly is bulging, and that can compromise the quality of your practice. Of course, if you attend an early-morning class and need a bite to eat beforehand, that's okay—just limit yourself to something small or light, such as a spoon of nut butter or half of an energy bar.

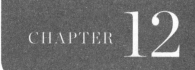

CHAPTER 12

Beautify Your Skin / Take Your Face into Your Healing Hands

WHAT DO WE ALL INSTINCTIVELY DO WHEN WE WALK PAST a window of an office building or a store at the mall? We check our reflections. Mirror, mirror, everywhere. Any shiny surface. We judge our own appearance at every opportunity.

We women are pretty tough on ourselves. And we scrutinize nothing with greater zeal than we do our own faces—and with good reason. Like it or not, we're being judged by the look of our skin by others, too.

As much as we'd all like to say that subtle signs of aging are no biggie, admit it, friends: Wrinkles and age spots can kill your confidence the same way that a few extra pounds can bring you down. Get this: In a study in *Aesthetic Surgery Journal,* women in their twenties cited their skin as a primary area they'd like to change. Can you believe it? Women in their twenties engaging in "old talk"? Dissatisfaction with skin rivals body dissatisfaction for many, many women.

Unfortunately, because it is exposed to the cruel world 24-7, your face is more vulnerable to wear and tear than other parts of your body. Fortunately, for the same reasons, it tends to be more resilient and responsive to some simple strategies to keep it healthy, supple, and smooth.

"New antiaging technologies keep popping up, but many aren't backed by science and may not do much more than a basic moisturizer," says Jeannette Graf, MD, an assistant clinical professor of dermatology at the Icahn School of Medicine at Mount Sinai Hospital.

Sounds like a bummer, but it's actually good news because it means that you can simplify your antiaging routine down to basic dermatology products and then do some deft makeup work to present yourself to the world with a confident glow. I like to stick with the products that are proven to work; sunscreen, coconut oil, argan oil, retinol, and peptides are at the top of my list. At age 44, I thankfully still get compliments on my skin—and I plan to keep it that way. You can, too.

What to Do

If you want to keep your skin looking beautiful and youthful (and who doesn't?), here are the basics that'll get the job done. There's nothing revolutionary here, but do you really do all of this religiously? Start to, and you'll see the difference.

BLOCK THE SUN

Reason number one to apply a generous coating of sunscreen and reapply frequently: It significantly reduces your risk of skin cancer—including the deadliest kind, melanoma. But my reasons for slathering the stuff on aren't just to prevent disease; there's a dose of vanity at work, too. Which brings me to reason number two: It prevents *photoaging,* or premature aging caused by the sun's UV rays. Listen to Whitney Bowe, MD, an assistant clinical professor of dermatology at SUNY Downstate Medical Center in New York: "UV breaks down collagen, which gives skin its strength and support—like scaffolding—and elastin, which makes skin plump. And when you're fair-skinned like I am, that breakdown happens even faster because your skin doesn't have pigment to protect it against damage from those UV rays."

Slather on sunscreen like it's butter on bread. Do it daily; don't skimp. In a 2013 study in *Annals of Internal Medicine,* people were asked to apply SPF 15 (or higher) sunscreen to their faces, necks, arms, and hands every morning and to reapply after showering, after spending significant time in the sun, and after sweating heavily. Another group was instructed to use sunscreen only as they saw fit. Four and a half years later, the researchers followed up with both groups, and here's what they found: The daily sunscreen users showed no detectable increase in signs of skin aging, such as wrinkles or dark spots. We guess the other group was pretty bummed.

The type of sunscreen you choose makes a difference. "Lotions tend to provide the best coverage because they're the thickest," says Katie Rodan, MD, a clinical assistant professor of dermatology at Stanford University School of Medicine. When it's time to reapply, you can reach for less labor-intensive formulas, such as solids and sprays. "Sticks are great for facial touch-ups because they offer so much control," says Karyn Grossman, MD, a dermatologist in Santa Monica, California, and New York City. "Sprays are good for the body because they're easy to apply, but you still have to spritz liberally—enough to initially see a white film on the skin—to get the appropriate SPF. A fine mist isn't going to fully cover you."

BE A SELECTIVE SCREENER

Low-SPF sunscreens offer little to no help against aging, cancer-causing UVA rays. That's why the FDA now requires any sunscreen under SPF 15 to state that it prevents sunburns only. Why is SPF 30 sunscreen—not the bottles with the crazy-high SPF—your sweet spot? "The sky-high numbers are mostly a marketing ploy," says Barbara Gilchrest, MD, professor and chair emeritus of the department of dermatology at Boston University School of Medicine. "People think they're doing themselves a favor by using sunscreen with a high SPF, but the difference is incremental." In other words, you don't need to spend extra money on SPF 50; go for SPF 30 and reapply frequently. Most important is making sure you're not using a bottle left over from that 2008 disaster in Key West with your ex. Most

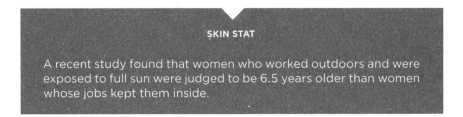

SKIN STAT

A recent study found that women who worked outdoors and were exposed to full sun were judged to be 6.5 years older than women whose jobs kept them inside.

sunscreens are designed to stay potent for up to 3 years, but that's assuming you didn't let them bake in the sun. "Leaving sunblock in intense heat for a prolonged amount of time may make it less effective," says Mitchel Chasin, MD, medical director of Reflections Center for Skin and Body in New Jersey.

DOUBLE YOUR DOSE

For proper protection, you need to apply a full ounce of sunscreen from head to toe—about the amount you'd need to fill up that souvenir shot glass from Cabo San Lucas. While you're at it, make it a double: "Most people use only one-third to half as much sunscreen as they should be using, and they apply it unevenly," says Steven Q. Wang, MD, director of dermatologic surgery at Memorial Sloan-Kettering Cancer Center. "If you apply two coats, theoretically you're going to put on more and deliver it more evenly." We know this might feel like a chore, but it's the best thing you can do to stay safe.

PROTECT YOURSELF YEAR-ROUND

Yes, even when the weather outside is frightful. Sun damage can occur in winter, too, even if you spend most of your time inside. If you sit near a window at work, for example, you're probably soaking up UVA rays because most windows don't filter out this type of ultraviolet radiation—the kind responsible for wrinkling, sagging, and leathery skin, according to the Skin Cancer Foundation.

USE YOUR SMARTPHONE TO SAVE YOUR SKIN

Setting a sunscreen alarm may sound a little overzealous, but if it will help you remember to protect your skin, it's totally worth it, right? In a recent *Archives of Dermatology* study, people who got daily reminders were almost twice as likely to apply sunscreen as those who weren't prompted. An alternative to setting an alarm: Simply make applying sunscreen a regular part of your morning routine, as something you always do right after you wash your face. If you still need an extra nudge, stick a note on your bathroom mirror.

COVER UP IN THE BUFF

To ensure that you hit every last spot (if you plan on being in the sun in a bathing suit or shorts), strip down to your birthday suit before you apply it. Ideally, this should happen 30 minutes before heading out for the day. Start on the right side of your body—arms, shoulders, legs, etc.—then move to the left side, zeroing in on your chest, stomach, and back along the way. Once that's done, go back to the right side and repeat the process. Make sure to hit the oft-overlooked areas: your hairline, behind your ears, your lips, and the backs of your hands, feet, and neck.

MOISTURIZE WITH COCONUT OIL BELOW THE NECK

Coconut oil—the organic kind—is the one moisturizer I consistently use on my body. It's all natural and capable of tackling even the toughest cases of dry skin. In fact, an *International Journal of Dermatology* study showed that rubbing on virgin coconut oil every day for 7 weeks boosted skin hydration by 32 percent in people with mild to moderate eczema. Bonus: The stuff smells divine, although you can get certain brands that are odorless, if you prefer.

To enjoy the greatest benefits:

Go virgin. The virgin variety really is worth the extra cash: It's extracted without using heat, whereas regular coconut oil is subjected to high temperatures during processing, which may wipe out some of the beneficial antioxidants and fatty acids, the study researchers say.

Oil up after a shower. This will help lock in the moisture on your skin, explains Francesca Fusco, MD, assistant clinical professor of dermatology at the Icahn School of Medicine at Mount Sinai Hospital. One word of caution: Make sure the coconut oil has dried completely before putting on your clothes, since it can stain fabric.

Pump up your body wash. You could buy a coconut oil–infused body wash—an easy way to add an extra dose of the stuff to your skin-care regimen—but why not make your own? Debra Jaliman, MD, a dermatologist in New York City, suggests adding a squirt of the stuff to your favorite bottle for a body wash with potent moisturizing power.

SAVE ARGAN OIL FOR YOUR FACE

I rarely use regular cream to moisturize my face—I'm all about the oils, particularly argan, which gives your skin the dewy glow that every woman seeks (and often loses with age). As we get older and our estrogen levels start to decline, our skin naturally becomes increasingly parched. "Your oil glands don't secrete as much as they did when you were younger," says Dr. Fusco. "As a result, your skin gets dryer."

INSTANT AGE ERASER

Rinse with Rice Water

Steal this antiaging secret from the East: Many women in China use rice water to cleanse their faces because rice has antioxidants that help prevent premature skin aging, says esthetician Christine Chin, owner of Christine Chin Spa in New York City. Give it a try: Soak Chinese rice (sold at Chinese grocery stores) in bottled water for 20 minutes. Strain out the rice, then dunk a washcloth in the water. Apply the damp cloth to your face for 10 minutes once a week.

ASK THE LIFE STYLIST

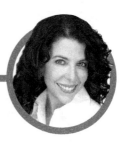

Francesca Fusco, MD, assistant clinical professor of dermatology at the Icahn School of Medicine at Mount Sinai Hospital

Q > Can I wear makeup with built-in SPF instead of sunscreen?

A < Don't cheat yourself out of good protection. A recent study from Memorial Sloan-Kettering Cancer Center found that most SPF-spiked beauty products skimp on the all-important UVA-blocking ingredients. If you're relying on a tinted mineral powder with SPF, it won't give you enough coverage unless you apply at least 10 times the normal amount—and then you'd just look orange. So think of your makeup as an extra layer of protection and always apply a lightweight, broad-spectrum sunscreen, too.

Q > Will applying oil to my face clog my pores?

A < If you slather olive oil straight from your kitchen onto your face, then yes, you're right to worry about the state of your pores. But if you use a product labeled specifically for the skin on your face, then it's a nongreasy formula that will only enhance—not compromise—your complexion.

Argan oil can help counteract that: In a 2013 study, postmenopausal
women who applied the oil every night experienced a significant increase in
the amount of moisture in their skin. The essential fatty acids nourish skin
cells, sealing in much-needed moisture by reinforcing your skin's top layer,
explains Dr. Graf. "If you buy an all-natural argan oil, you avoid putting
chemicals on your skin," adds Dr. Fusco. But that's not the only way argan
oil fights the ravages of time: This Moroccan miracle-worker is packed with
polyphenols, a class of compounds known to ward off wrinkles caused by
sun damage, according to a study review in the *European Journal of Lipid
Science and Technology.*

I tend to have dry skin, but even blemish-prone people can benefit
from the slick stuff because argan oil helps control the release of sebum,
the waxy substance secreted by your skin. In fact, a study in the *Journal of
Cosmetic Dermatology* found that an argan oil–infused cream combated
facial greasiness and improved the overall appearance of oily skin.

To enjoy the greatest benefits:

Apply it over night cream. If your skin is extremely dry, pair
argan oil and a moisturizing night cream for extra p.m.
protection against a flaking face. After applying the cream,
simply pat a few drops of argan oil all over your forehead,
nose, cheeks, and chin to lock in the moisturizer. Try Josie
Maran Argan Oil.

Or use it alone. Oily complexion? Skip the night cream, and use
only argan oil as your evening moisturizer, patting it evenly
across your face.

UNDO THE DAMAGE

Sunscreen shields your skin from future trouble. But how can you handle
the damage that's already been done? One word: retinol. This form of vitamin A is the most powerful over-the-counter ingredient for softening
lines and firming skin over time. In fact, there are decades' worth of data

supporting its ability to reduce wrinkles and fade spots. In one *Journal of Cosmetic Dermatology* study, women who used a retinol product showed improvements in fine lines, wrinkles, skin firmness and evenness, and clarity of complexion after as little as 2 weeks. "Retinol regulates the cell turnover of your skin," says Dr. Fusco. Read: It makes sure your skin cells reproduce, so you avoid the dull appearance of dead cell buildup and eradicate, or at least fade, brown spots.

Unlike most of the stuff women smear on their faces, retinol is actually able to penetrate past your skin's surface, so it truly targets the extracellular matrix, where collagen and elastin reside, according to the *Journal of Clinical Investigation.* Once deep inside your skin, retinol enhances the production of fibroblasts, the cells responsible for manufacturing collagen, says Dr. Fusco. "That improves the appearance of fine lines and wrinkles."

To enjoy the greatest benefits:

Start slowly. Retinol is pretty powerful stuff, so you should start off using it just once or twice a week, to avoid irritation. If no peeling, redness, or flakiness occurs after a month, you can slowly increase your frequency of usage. For example, try using it three times a week (every other day). Then, after another month, increase to four times a week, then to five at the 2-month mark, and so on.

IS A OKAY?

You may have heard reports that vitamin A, an ingredient in many sunscreens, may be a cancer risk. The studies that exposed this possibility were performed on rats exposed to exceptionally high doses that one would not typically get through regular use. The FDA has not changed its guidelines for use of vitamin A in sunscreen. If you wish to avoid sunscreens that include vitamin A, consider products using its derivatives retinol and retinyl palmitate.

Apply it strategically. "Never apply it to a freshly washed or exfoliated face or on your eyelids," says Dr. Fusco. "Never apply more than what the product label tells you to, and never use it when you're going to be exposed to a lot of sunlight." So if you're going sailing on Saturday, skip your Friday-night retinol regimen. Dr. Fusco also suggests that you start with the lowest percentage of retinol to see how your skin reacts, noting that 1 percent retinol is very strong.

Find your formula. I like Retriderm Serum Plus by Biopelle (0.75 percent retinol), but it's important to choose the right serum for your skin type.

- Oily or acne-prone: Your thicker skin can withstand a strong dose of retinol, so go for the highest over-the-counter strength available (1 percent)—for example, SkinCeuticals Retinol 1.0.

- Dry: To avoid irritation, look for a product with a cream base, like RoC Retinol Correxion Sensitive Night Cream.

- Sensitive: Opt for retinaldehyde, a kinder, gentler version of the chemical that converts to retinoic acid at a deeper skin level, dodging surface irritation. Try Eau Thermale Avène Rétrinal+ 0.05 Cream.

TIGHTEN UP WITH A PEPTIDE

Peptides are chains of amino acids and proteins that have been shown to boost your complexion in a variety of ways. Some are matrix metalloproteinase inhibitors, which means they block compounds that break down collagen, says Dr. Fusco. "Peptides—like retinols—improve collagen but won't cause irritation," adds Paul Jarrod Frank, MD, a clinical assistant professor of dermatology at NYU Medical Center. "Combining them with retinols can offer a gentle but effective antiaging boost." There's also Argireline, a synthetic peptide with a Botox-like effect. And there are still other peptides that hydrate, and some that decrease puffing.

To enjoy the greatest benefits:

Choose right. Instead of focusing on ingredient names, read the box and pick the one for the problem you have. For example, if you're looking for a collagen-boosting peptide, scan for the words "firming" or "lifting." One warning: If you're targeting the skin under your eyes, make sure the label says the product is specifically formulated for that area. The skin around your eyes is sensitive and needs special treatment.

THE COOLEST TOOL FOR CLEAR SKIN

My skin-care routine may be simple, but I still know when it's time to bring out the big guns. My go-to tool for serious cleansing is a rotating facial brush. These revved-up rotators, like the Clarisonic, Olay Pro-X Advanced Cleansing System, or Neutrogena Wave Sonic, go where hands alone cannot: deep into your pores to remove every trace of dirt and makeup. "It's so much easier to control the level of abrasion you get with a brush than with an acid or scrub, plus it's gentle enough for people with sensitive skin," says Anne Chapas, MD, an assistant clinical professor of dermatology at New York University.

Sloughing off the top layer of dead cells creates an immediate radiance, but there are long-term benefits, too. Eliminating all that pore-clogging gunk allows antiaging creams and serums to penetrate deeper and, therefore, work better. Ready to power up your complexion? Start on the lowest setting, holding the brush very lightly against your skin, and use a mild, gentle cleanser.

Supplement with makeup. Blush, foundation, and eye shadow can do more than pretty you up. They can also smooth out wrinkles and uneven texture with peptides that are normally relegated to antiaging skin treatments. And while these makeup items can't replace your daily skin-care regimen, "the extra dose of antiagers they provide helps you achieve better results in both the short and long term," says Dr. Fusco. Here are a few to check out for various reasons.

- You want to firm up your face: Fusion Beauty Colorceuticals Sculptdiva Contouring and Sculpting Blush is a cream blush made with collagen-stimulating peptides that plump cheeks for a firmer look.

- You want to tighten your lips and lids: Aveda Nourish-Mint Lip Definer contains collagen-boosting peptides that make lips appear fuller. Babor Super Soft Eye Shadow tightens lids with peptide-based firming agents typically found in antiaging eye creams.

The Skin-Care Plan

This daily routine capitalizes on the tiny biological changes your body experiences around the clock, giving you opportunities to boost your beauty potential throughout the day. In essence, you are cycling your regimen around your internal clock and the state of your skin at key times during the day. The following is an antiaging game plan suggested by Dr. Fusco.

YOUR SKIN-CARE SHOPPING LIST

❏ Nonfoaming facial
cleanser

❏ Caffeinated eye gel

❏ Baking soda or sugar

❏ Virgin coconut oil

❏ SPF 30 sunscreen

❏ Moisturizing face
spray (optional)

❏ Textured facial
cleansing wipes

❏ Exfoliating facial scrub

❏ Rotating facial brush
(optional)

❏ Retinol-based product

❏ Night cream
(containing glycerin or
hyaluronic acid and
peptides; optional)

❏ Argan oil formulated
for facial skin

❏ Peptide-based eye
cream

❏ Nutrient-rich hand and
foot mask

THE MORNING ROUTINE

Moisture gets sucked out of your skin and lips while you're sleeping, and
what's left hanging around tends to pool in the most unfortunate places—
around your eyes, where skin is thinner and more delicate. Around 4 a.m.
your temperature, blood pressure, and hormone levels begin to rise,
boosting oiliness. This adds a bit of hydration, but you still need to help your
skin along by taking the following steps.

1. Your skin hasn't accumulated much filth overnight, so you don't
need to scour your face come morning. You can do as little as
splash water on your face, but if you want to freshen up, use a
moisturizing, nonfoaming cleanser. It will remove any impurities
while also hydrating your skin. It's best to use something that
doesn't foam, because the ingredients that make cleansers foamy
tend to strip the skin and irritate it.

2. To depuff your eyes, Dr. Fusco recommends storing a caffeinated eye gel in the fridge and dabbing it on first thing in the morning. "The coldness and caffeine act as vasoconstrictors, and they'll pull the puff right out," she says. Try First Aid Beauty Detox Eye Roller, rolling from the outer to inner corner of each eye.

3. Sprinkle baking soda or sugar on a toothbrush and gently buff your lips to remove dry, flaky skin and reveal a smooth kisser.

4. Shower, blot your skin dry, and apply coconut oil all over your body.

5. Twenty to 30 minutes before you head out, slather a grape-size blob of SPF 30 sunscreen on your face. (If you're going to be outside all day, apply a larger amount all over your body or, at the very least, on the exposed areas of your body.) Hint: You can mix your sunscreen with your foundation to create a tinted blend.

LAYER IT ON

If you're like most women, you have an arsenal of face products that you use daily—but even the best beautifiers won't reach their full potential if you layer them the wrong way. Apply from lightest (or thinnest) to heaviest (or thickest) to make sure each ingredient can be absorbed into your skin, and wait 2 to 3 minutes between layers so you don't dilute them. Here's a breakdown.

Step 1: Liquids, like toners or astringents

Step 2: Serums, gels, or anything translucent

Step 3: Moisturizing lotions

Step 4: Eye creams

Step 5: Sunscreen, regardless of consistency

Step 6: Makeup (if you wear it)

THE LATE-AFTERNOON TOUCH-UP

Your body starts slowly shifting gears again around 4 p.m. Your body temperature cools and your blood pressure lowers, causing you (and your skin) to look drained and sleepy. To breathe life back into your complexion, spritz on a light moisturizing face spray; the cooling blast of hydration will be energizing. Some sprays—like Sircuit Cosmeceuticals Molecular Mist+—contain skin-healthy antioxidants that block free radicals from damaging your skin. "Any use of antioxidants will aid in the antiaging toolbox," says Dr. Fusco.

THE NIGHTTIME ROUTINE

While you're getting your beauty sleep, your body is hard at work, repairing weakened muscle fibers and regenerating skin cells. Because night is your body's prime recovery time, a big chunk of your 24-hour routine should be focused here.

1. Start with textured cleansing wipes, like Aveeno Positively Radiant Daily Cleansing Pads, Pond's Luminous Clean Wet Cleansing Towelettes, or Simple Radiance textured cleansing facial wipes. They'll cut through the day's grime, oil, and sunscreen and gently exfoliate your skin at the same time. "These are extremely hygienic, since you use them, then throw them out," says Dr. Fusco. "And they're safe to use all over your face."

2. Twice a week, go for a deeper cleanse. Use either a physical scrub (one that contains exfoliating beads) or a chemical scrub (one with salicylic acid, alpha hydroxy acid, or glycolic acid) to rid your skin of dulling dead-cell buildup. "If your skin is super sensitive or develops broken blood vessels very easily, use a chemical scrub," Dr. Fusco advises. "If your skin is oily and you have large pores, a physical scrub will plump the skin up around your pores, making them appear smaller." Buff gently with a circular motion, using either a face towel or a rotating brush (see page 195) to apply your cleanser. If you're using a brush and your skin type requires a physical scrub, stick to one with synthetic, rather than natural, beads. Natural exfoliants, such as apricot seeds, have jagged edges that could tear your skin with the power of a rotating brush behind them.

AGE-PROOFING BELOW THE NECK

In a recent survey, 67 percent of women admitted to focusing their antiaging efforts only on their faces. But, hello, the skin on the rest of your body gets old, too! Here's how to do a little damage control.

Chest

Décolletage skin is thin and delicate, making it the below-the-neck part most prone to sun damage and wrinkles. Dermatologist Cheryl Karcher, MD, suggests smoothing on a collagen-stimulating retinol like RoC Retinol Correxion Deep Wrinkle Night Cream at night.

Hands

Slather your antiaging facial cream on your mitts. While specialized creams may claim to target different areas of the body, the active ingredients in antiaging formulas are the same, says New York City dermatologist David Colbert, MD. The retinoids (such as Retin-A) that promote cell turnover and stimulate collagen (which is responsible for skin's firmness) on your face can do the same for your hands. Another option: a hydrating, skin-brightening hand cream, like Avon Anew Clinical Absolute Even Spot Correcting Hand Cream with SPF 15. It moisturizes with dimethicone, fades discoloration with phytol, and protects against sun damage.

Arms and Legs

Look for a hydrator that also exfoliates and reduces inflammation (read: redness), another side effect of aging that's common on the limbs, says Fredric Brandt, MD, a dermatologist in New York City. SkinCeuticals Body Retexturing Treatment contains hyaluronic acid to boost moisture and niacinamide to zap inflammation. Use it once a day in the morning.

Feet

A cream spiked with lactic acid will slough off dead skin, leaving feet looking and feeling baby soft, says Dr. Karcher. Try Eucerin Intensive Repair Extra-Enriched Foot Creme. Apply daily.

3. After washing and drying your face (hint: use a fresh towel every evening), wait 10 to 20 minutes before slathering on a retinol-based product. (See page 192 for help finding one for your skin type.) "This will accelerate cell turnover, which evens out pigmentation and increases collagen production," says Dr. Fusco.

4. If you have very dry skin, apply a night cream next. Look for one that contains glycerin or hyaluronic acid (to protect against moisture loss) and peptides, such as Vichy Aqualia Thermal Serum or Vichy LiftActiv Serum. Spread the serum between your hands, then gently massage it onto your face. "Hyaluronic acid absorbs and holds on to moisture," says Dr. Fusco.

5. Smooth on argan oil, choosing a bottle labeled specifically for facial skin. Squeeze a pea-size amount into your palm, rub your hands together, and pat the oil all over your face. This will seal in your night moisturizer or, if you didn't use a cream, will combat dryness on its own.

6. Pat an eye cream with peptides over crow's-feet and brow bones and under your eyes to firm and tighten the skin.

7. Once a week, apply a nutrient-rich mask to your hands and feet, and wear cotton gloves and socks overnight. Try OPI Manicure Pedicure White Tea Mask. And on either a weekly or monthly basis, coat your hair and scalp in an oil-based mask, such as Clear Scalp and Hair Intense Hydration Deep Nourishing Mask.

THREE TAKEAWAYS TO TRY TODAY

1. **Set an alarm on your smartphone to remind you to reapply sunscreen,** especially during the off-season months when you don't normally think about it.

2. **Moisturize your face with argan oil,** which is loaded with age-erasing polyphenols.

3. **Eat some sun protection.** Start a 10-week effort to boost your lycopene intake by eating more watermelon and tomatoes, rich sources of the antioxidant.

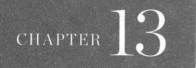
Erase Years with Makeup/Ways to Enhance Your Unique Assets

CAN THE RIGHT MAKEUP REALLY TURN BACK TIME? You bet! It all comes down to a skillful artistic endeavor called creating contrast. In a recent study, scientists at Gettysburg College tweaked the tones of facial skin in photos of women 20 to 70 years old, then asked volunteers to estimate the age of each woman. Those with minimal contrast—a monochromatic appearance, with little color difference in the lips, eye area, and skin—looked the oldest. Makes sense, since with each passing birthday our lips, lashes, and eyebrows naturally lighten. So creating contrast is one way to turn back time and enhance the beauty of your bone structure. Makeup, as you know, is also a godsend for masking the kinds of little flaws that drive us nuts. And used wisely and minimally, it can draw the viewer's eye to our most appealing, youthful features while de-emphasizing the markers of, um, experience, wisdom, and yes, the years.

Now, the antiaging effects of makeup don't have to be dramatic. In fact, they shouldn't be: *Too much* contrast can look heavy and put an even brighter spotlight on your fine lines and wrinkles. Just as with my skin-care routine, I prefer to keep my makeup simple: I stick to the same basic look almost every day. Even for special occasions, my "splurge" is just a little extra eye shadow and a nail color that pops. Why? Because I've figured out what works—and by that, I mean what keeps me looking youthful: mascara, berry-colored lips, cream blush, and a liquid highlighter. What'll work for you? It'll take some experimenting, but that's where the fun begins. Try playing around with these subtle ways to tint your face . . . right back to your baby-faced years.

Turn Back the Clock on Your . . .

COMPLEXION

Go for a creamy, luminous foundation that matches the skin on your lower cheeks. Don't go by your neck: Since it's been mostly shaded from the sun all these years, it may be much lighter, says New York City makeup artist Erica Whelan. Divide an almond-size amount over cheeks, forehead, nose, and chin, and then blend with a damp sponge for a light veil of coverage that diffuses the look of any fine lines.

Also, be strategic with bronzer. The last thing sun-spotted skin needs is a coating of brown powder. But if you crave a golden glow, "sweep a

---

INSTANT AGE ERASER

Wear Lavender

When your eyes look whiter, the surrounding skin looks brighter. "Lavender is one of my go-to eye-shadow colors for adding sparkle and counteracting red tones in your whites and the skin around your eyes," says Lori Taylor, a global makeup artist for Smashbox cosmetics. Dust opalescent lavender shadow over your lids, and pair it with deep-black mascara.

light-tan bronzer along the very top of your hairline and your temples, swinging the brush under your cheekbones, as if you're making a C-shape," says Sandy Linter, a New York City makeup artist. "You'll enhance bone structure and also make the rest of your face seem lighter."

EYELIDS AND LASHES

Even your lashes are subject to the hormonal fluctuations of aging. "When estrogen and progesterone start to drop in our thirties, lashes can become thinner," says Doris Day, MD, a clinical professor of dermatology at New York University. "This hormonal change can slow regrowth, so you're no longer replacing what you've lost." Daily lash curling and harsh makeup removal are also to blame, since this constant abuse can scar the follicles so the hairs no longer grow back.

Fading and thinning make your lash lines so faint that you have to squint to see 'em. That's why one of the best look-younger-now eye tricks is to reinforce the lash line, says New York City and Los Angeles makeup artist Sarah Tanno. Step one: Pick a pencil eyeliner. Its sharp edge allows for precision, lets you get very close to your lash line (for a natural effect), and offers more control than gels and liquid liners do. Try espresso on light skin and black on medium or dark.

When you're ready to apply liner, pull the outer corner of your top eyelid taut, then wiggle the pencil in between your lashes. Wing the liner slightly upward as you reach the outer corner: "Old eyes tilt downward, and if you follow the curve, you'll just look sad," says Linter. Skip liner below—it can drag your eyes down.

Dust a light-to-medium bronze eye shadow into your creases, then place a champagne hue on your lids, right up to the bronze. Redefining your eye socket and highlighting your lids helps combat the appearance of sagging, droopy lids. Coat your lashes with a primer, which creates a long, lush appearance, then double up: Apply two coats of black mascara, followed by two coats of brown. The combination can help boost depth and dimension.

MAKEUP STYLISTS' BEST TRICKS

Antiaging skin-care products can take weeks to show results, but these makeup secrets will help in one quick stroke of a brush.

The Problem: Undereye circles

The Fix: Rub a concealer brush in a pot of orange-based concealer (orange neutralizes the purple and blue tones of dark circles), says Martin Maulawizada, a makeup artist and global artistry director for Laura Mercier. Working from the inner corners of your eyes out, brush over dark areas; if darkness still shows through, apply an extra coat. Try Benefit Erase Paste in Medium.

The Problem: Acne

The Fix: A yellow-based concealer will cut the redness and help the pimple fade into the surrounding skin. Using a concealer brush, apply a dot the size of the blemish directly on top of it, and blend the color out and around the mark; tap translucent powder on top to set the concealer. Try Physicians Formula Youthful Wear Cosmeceutical Youth-Boosting Concealer.

The Problem: Crow's-feet

The Fix: You should avoid concealer and "spackle"-type products. "These would help if you didn't smile or move your face at all," says Maulawizada. "The less texture you put on wrinkles, the better they look." What can you use? A brightening serum to reflect light in a softer way. Try Laura Mercier Flawless Skin Repair Eye Serum.

The Problem: Rosacea

The Fix: Dip your ring finger into a yellow-based camouflage, and then lightly tap over the patch of rosacea until the redness has disappeared.

The Problem: Dark spots

The Fix: Use a concealer brush to dab orange-based cover-up onto a spot and blend by lightly tapping with your ring finger. Repeat until the spot is invisible, and set with translucent powder.

CHEEKS

The natural flush that once graced your face now emerges only after you run a 5-K. To fake it all day, every day, "look for formulas and shades that help energize and add sheen," says Whelan. Reach for a cream or gel blush: Thanks to their dewy finish, they bring a youthful, fresh glow back to your skin. If you have light or medium skin, opt for a light or midtone pinky apricot; if you're dark-skinned, go for a raspberry hue.

What *not* to copy from your younger years? Placement. "We're told to put blush on our apples, but as we age, our skin sags and nasolabial folds [the creases that run from your nose to the outer corners of your mouth] become more pronounced," warns Whelan. "Putting blush close to the center of your face draws more attention there. The answer is to redirect: Find the highest point of your cheekbones—about an inch directly below your eye's outer corner—and dab blush right below that point, blending toward your hairline. Then apply a pea-size dab of pink liquid highlighter on the highest point of your cheekbones, using a light tapping motion with the tip of your finger. Try Make Up For Ever Uplight Face Luminizer Gel. Emphasizing your cheekbones while strategically applying blush to avoid the hollow-cheeked look that comes with age gives you a youthful, feminine look.

LIPS

Over time, lips get smaller and paler, and their borders start to become less defined. Plus, the aging process causes a loss of bone density, which "makes our faces appear sunken and provides even less support to the lips, forcing

INSTANT AGE ERASER

Sip through a Straw

Teeth darken with age because they absorb color from foods and drinks. Using a straw will keep staining enemies like tea, coffee, and soda off your teeth, says Nancy Rosen, DMD, a cosmetic dentist.

them to roll inward and look thinner," adds Macrene Alexiades-Armenakas, MD, PhD, an assistant professor of dermatology at Yale School of Medicine. Great news, right?

I'm not a huge fan of lip liner, but if your kisser is looking too lean, it can help. Reinstate your lips' shape by tracing them with a pencil in a shade that closely matches their middle, then fill them in. Hint: Apply your lipstick with a brush so you can get into every corner and edge. What color is right for you? A medium rose is pretty on light to medium skin. If your complexion is dark, try red-toned plum; top with a matching sheer, moisturizing lipstick—adding sheen helps visually plump up the lips a bit, especially when it's placed in the center of the lower lip.

How will this refresh your face? Yet again, it all comes down to contrast. In another British study, women whose lips were a different color from their skin—specifically, a shade of red—were seen as more feminine and attractive. That may be because brighter lips reflect higher estrogen levels, a sign of youth and fertility. Plus, women with fuller-looking lips are perceived as younger, according to another British study.

TEETH

No matter how perfect your makeup, your smile has a way of drawing attention away from the rest of your features. Teeth are the brightest, most visual feature on your face—or at least they should be. Your choppers can make you look older or younger, depending on how well you care for them.

With age, the outermost layer of tooth enamel thins and exposes the inner dentin, which has a yellowish hue. "That's why we associate white teeth with youthfulness," says Jason Olitsky, DDS, a cosmetic dentist in Ponte Vedra Beach, Florida. Smoking and consuming food or drink that would stain your clothes contribute to this natural discoloration over time, especially if you don't brush immediately afterward.

So how can you turn back time? Strips are the most potent whiteners at the drugstore—they create a suction cup effect that doesn't allow saliva to get underneath and dilute the bleaching agent. For yellowing, try Crest 3D White Intensive Professional Effects Whitestrips, which have an extra-thick layer of peroxide and can give you the sparkling results you'd get from a dentist. If your teeth are sensitive or just need a minor touch-up, use strips with a lower level of peroxide, like Crest 3D White Gentle Routine Whitestrips.

Don't whiten more than twice a year, as overdoing it can make your teeth look weirdly translucent. Not sure how white is white enough? Look to your eyes as a guide to your ideal shade. "Your teeth and the whites of your eyes should match," says Emanuel Layliev, a cosmetic dentist in New York City. Maintain results by brushing with a whitening fluoride toothpaste daily. Rembrandt Deeply White + Peroxide Fresh Mint Toothpaste is a dentist favorite.

If your stains are more brown than yellow, see your dentist for Philips Zoom Whitening, which takes about an hour and costs roughly $500. Unfortunately, not even the most intense whitening treatment tackles grayness—this issue requires veneers, which are sheets of ceramic bonded to each tooth at a cost of $1,000 to $3,000 per tooth.

THREE TAKEAWAYS TO TRY TODAY

1. **Reinforce your lash lines** with espresso or black to make your eyes look brighter.

2. **Never use a spackle-style concealer** around the eyes because it will make crow's feet look cakey.

3. **Use an over-the-counter tooth whitener** to do more to make you look youthful than any amount of makeup.

INSTANT AGE ERASER

Give Your Smile a Boost

It's Color Wheel 101: Cool blue is opposite warm yellow, so they nullify each other. For a quick fix, Luster Now! Instant Whitening Toothpaste "deposits a temporary blue tint, making teeth appear whiter for hours," says cosmetic chemist Jim Hammer.

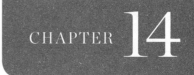

CHAPTER 14

Bring Back the Bounce and Body/

Baby Your Hair to Coax Out
Shine and Fullness

YOUR HAIR AGES RIGHT ALONG WITH THE REST OF YOU—and I'm not just talking about the grays that start peeking out around your 40th birthday. Paradi Mirmirani, MD, a dermatologist in Vallejo, California, who specializes in hair disorders, shared this wonderful news with me: "Every year, the diameter of our hair strands gets thinner, we have fewer hairs in the growth phase, and hair grows at a slower rate." At the same time, the chemicals and heat we've been using for years catch up with us.

It's no surprise, then, that your hair may start exhibiting a rougher, drier texture, and you may start to notice hair loss or thinning. "Hair is a fiber, like wool. It can only take so much wear and tear," says Dr. Mirmirani. The good news it that your scalp is one of the easiest places to rejuvenate: The right cut, color, and products can instantly restore your locks' former sheen and add movement that makes you look years younger. You can do a lot to protect and serve your hair, just as you do with your skin. Try these strategies.

Turn Back the Clock

ADD DIMENSION

Covering your grays with color isn't an automatic fix for aging up top. You're not painting a wall. Too much contrast or not enough dimension can make you look washed out and older, says colorist Rita Hazan of New York City's Rita Hazan Salon. Fair-skinned brunette? Lighten hair one shade, then add caramel highlights. Blondes and reds: Go warm! Switch cool platinum streaks for golden ones, or weave in coppery pieces instead of cherry or burgundy, which aren't as face-flattering as you age.

LIGHTEN UP

Sporting an Elvira shade doesn't do your face any favors. You're better off lightening up, especially if you have naturally dark hair—it will make your skin appear to have more pigment so you don't look washed out. "As all of us get older, our skin becomes more sallow and our hair grows darker," says colorist Michael Canabe. "What makes you look younger is going back to the color you had as a kid. It warms up the skin and is instantly youthful."

GO LONG

Just because you're 45 doesn't mean it's time for a cropped mom 'do. "As you grow older, it's important to keep the softness in your hair and have some length to frame your face," says Oribe, a celebrity hairstylist. But keep in mind: Although long hair has no age limit, it does have rules. "Long, blunt hair can drag down the face and become aging," says celebrity stylist Richard Marin. "Layers lift and awaken the face, making you look younger." So ask your stylist to cut long layers all around and then face-framing ones no shorter than your chin—and keep just the back blunt. More bulk on the bottom prevents thin hair from looking scraggly.

DODGE DANDRUFF

The one accessory you should never sport: white flakes on your shoulders. The snowstorm on your sweater isn't always true dandruff, though, which is caused by a yeastlike fungus: It could just be a severe case of dry scalp. Like the skin on your body, your scalp gets flaky when it's parched. Your root Rx: Start by doing a hot oil treatment once a week, after shampooing and towel-drying your hair. Microwave ¼ cup of jojoba oil for 20 seconds, then dab a cotton ball into the oil and press it over your entire scalp. Wrap your hair in a towel for 20 minutes, then shampoo again, condition, and rinse as you normally would. If that doesn't soothe your scalp, you most likely have actual dandruff. In that case, switch to a medicated shampoo containing zinc pyrithione (the active ingredient in Garnier Fructis Anti-Dandruff Shampoo and many other dandruff shampoos), which will kill the fungus and stop the itching and flakes.

INSTANT AGE ERASER

Update Your Bangs

If you're over 35, pin-straight blunt-cut bangs can look too harsh and are horribly aging. Try this styling trick: While your bangs are clean and damp, blast them with a blow-dryer as you brush them repeatedly to one side, then to the other side, with an oval brush (a round one will make bangs puff up). This will tame any bends or pesky cowlicks, making your bangs fall gracefully. When your hair is dry, mist your bangs with a lightweight hair spray like Oribe Superfine Hair Spray.

KNOW YOUR HAIR TYPE

In your early twenties, your hair may have been able to withstand any product you slapped on it. But if you hope to preserve the shininess of your youth, it's wise to know your hair type and which specific products are right for it. Hair isn't just oily or dry—it's categorized by three characteristics: porosity (how much moisture it can hold), elasticity (how easily it breaks), and texture (how thick it is). This equation takes into account the hair you were born with, plus what you've done to it (color, blow-dry, style, etc.).

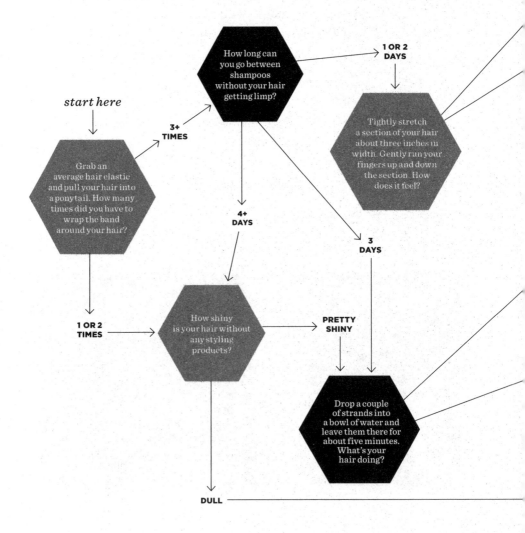

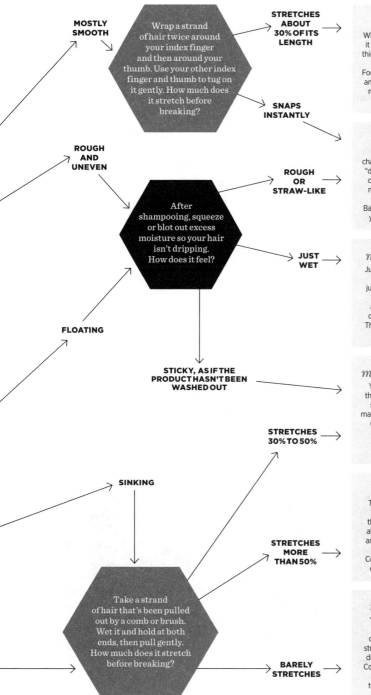

MOSTLY SMOOTH

Wrap a strand of hair twice around your index finger and then around your thumb. Use your other index finger and thumb to tug on it gently. How much does it stretch before breaking?

STRETCHES ABOUT 30% OF ITS LENGTH

SNAPS INSTANTLY

fine + healthy

What your hair has in healthiness, it lacks in volume. Each strand is thin and can't hold its own against certain hair-care ingredients. Focus on tress-plumping products and avoid heavy ones, which will make hair fall flat within hours of styling.

ROUGH AND UNEVEN

After shampooing, squeeze or blot out excess moisture so your hair isn't dripping. How does it feel?

ROUGH OR STRAW-LIKE

JUST WET

fine + damaged

While achieving fullness is a challenge for all skinny strands, the "damaged" part of your equation creates a double whammy: You need to find repairing products that don't make hair go limp. Balance volume and moisture and you'll restore your hair's luster.

medium + healthy

Just call you Goldilocks—not too much hair, not too little, but just right (and in fab condition). That means no ingredients are off limits, and any haircut or style you want is attainable. The goal is to keep your locks as pristine as they are now.

FLOATING

STICKY, AS IF THE PRODUCT HASN'T BEEN WASHED OUT

medium + damaged

Your strands are thick enough that any hairstyle works, but not so thick that they're tough to manage. The problem? Overstyling (or coloring) has caused split ends, frizz, and dullness. Strengthen with protein and you'll prevent breakage.

STRETCHES 30% TO 50%

SINKING

thick + healthy

There's an irony to fat strands: Their wide diameter makes them voluminous and sexy but also potentially coarser, frizzier, and less shiny than their thinner counterparts. Your mission: Condition! Hydrated thick hair is easier to style and less poufy.

STRETCHES MORE THAN 50%

Take a strand of hair that's been pulled out by a comb or brush. Wet it and hold at both ends, then pull gently. How much does it stretch before breaking?

BARELY STRETCHES

thick + damaged

Your hair is hard to control as is. Throw in lots of blow-drying, flat-ironing, dyeing, or straightening, and no wonder it's disobeying like a petulant child. Coddle it with mega moisturizers and mega frizz fighters. And try to use heat tools sparingly.

FINE AND HEALTHY

What your hair has in healthiness, it lacks in volume. Each strand is thin and can't hold its own against certain hair-care ingredients. Focus on tress-plumping products and avoid heavy ones, which will make your hair fall flat within hours of styling.

SHAMPOO: Do it every day. Sebum, dirt, and sweat buildup can make hair lifeless and can increase shedding and thinning. What kind of shampoo works best for you? Look for words like thickening, volumizing, or amplifying and ingredients like natural cellulose and polymers (both add bulk by filling in the space between strands). "Go for a shampoo that's translucent—opaque formulas generally have more intense ingredients, which may interfere with volume," says Jeni Thomas, a senior scientist at Procter & Gamble. Try Bumble and Bumble Thickening Shampoo.

CONDITIONER: Don't skip it, but only apply it to your ends. Ingredients to look for: cetrimonium chloride, cyclomethicone, and glycerin detangle and add lightweight hydration without any drag, says cosmetic chemist Perry Romanowksi. Avoid dimethicone and behentrimonium methosulfate, which make fine hair greasy. A smart place to start? Aveeno Pure Renewal Conditioner.

STYLERS: Anything creamy or waxy—especially if it contains beeswax or candelilla wax—will make your hair look flatter than a MacBook Air. To plump, go for a thickening spray containing

INSTANT AGE ERASER

Gloss Your Locks

A hair gloss, at home or in the salon, has sheen enhancers that coat the hair's cuticle and give the illusion of healthier hair, says colorist Sharon Dorram, owner of Sharon Dorram Color at Sally Hershberger in New York City. While the gloss sets, blast your head with a blow-dryer for even better results.

polyethylene particles, nylon, polyquaternium, or panthenol, such as Umberto Beverly Hills Volumizer Thickening Spray. Mist it onto damp palms and work from your roots out toward the ends of your strands. If it's texture and swing you seek, use a mousse like Herbal Essences Totally Twisted Curl Boosting Mousse. Smooth flyaways and add shine with a lightweight serum or spray containing oil— for example, Organix Nourishing Coconut Oil Weightless Hydrating Oil Mist.

FINE AND DAMAGED

While achieving fullness is a challenge for all skinny strands, the "damaged" part of your equation creates a double whammy: You need to find repairing products that don't make hair go limp. Balance volume and moisture, and you'll restore your hair's luster.

SHAMPOO: Choose one based on the state of your scalp: It's oily if your roots get greasy within a day of washing; it's dry if it feels tight or irritated and has occasional flakes. Oily scalps benefit from a gentle shampoo—that is, one without sulfates or sodium chloride, such as Alterna Bamboo Abundant Volume Shampoo. Dry scalp? Zinc pyrithione or carrot extract will prevent flaking and itching. Try Yes to Carrots Scalp Relief Shampoo.

CONDITIONER: Look for a bottle labeled *repairing, smoothing,* or *moisturizing* to revive your tortured locks. Ingredients to seek include glycerin (which softens rough edges in a nonweighty way), pomegranate oil (a light shine booster), hydrolyzed elastin (for flexibility), and peptides or wheat or oat protein (to strengthen), says hairstylist Nuri Yurt, who owns Toka Salon and Day Spa in Washington, DC. A product that fits the bill: Phyto Phytokératine Reparative Conditioning Treatment. What to avoid? Conditioners that contain dimethicone or behentrimonium methosulfate—they're too heavy for your hair.

AFTER YOUR SHOWER, tame and soften with a spray-on conditioner that contains cyclopentasiloxane, such as Garnier Fructis

Triple Nutrition Nutrient Spray for Dry, Damaged Hair. Mist it over the damaged areas. Deep-condition once a week with a mask laced with kernel oil or wheat-germ oil. Try Moroccanoil Weightless Hydrating Mask. Before shampooing, apply it to the bottom half of dry hair for 15 minutes.

STYLERS: A spray with nylon, polyethylene particles, or polyquaternium—such as Pureology Pure Volume Thickening Spray—beefs up fine hair like a protein shake bolsters weak muscles. Mist it onto your fingers and rake them through the top inch of your hair, then blow-dry upside down. Hint: Use a plastic-bristle brush, which will smooth without stretching your strands, says Tippi Shorter, a hairstylist in New York City. Steer clear of any alcohol-based styling products, since they'll further dry out your hair.

MEDIUM AND HEALTHY

We'll just call you Goldilocks—not too much hair, not too little, but just right (and in fab condition). That means no ingredients are off-limits and any haircut or style you want is attainable. The goal is to keep your locks as pristine as they are now.

SHAMPOO: Wash every other day with a formula geared for your scalp. If your roots get greasy fast, you're oily; fruit acids will nix grease and product buildup. If your scalp feels tight or irritated or you have occasional flaking, you're dry; hydrating babassu, olive, or sesame seed oil will help. In either case, you also want wheat or oat protein to retain your hair's resiliency. For an oily scalp, try Redken Hair Cleansing Cream Shampoo. For a dry scalp, try Fekkai Brilliant Glossing Shampoo.

CONDITIONER: For straight hair, stearalkonium chloride, a not-too-heavy plant-based fatty acid, offers antistatic benefits. The Cream by Paul Mitchell does the trick. If you have waves or curls, look for a blend of smoothing keratin protein and behentrimonium chloride, a waxier conditioner that helps tame tangles. Try Suave Professionals Keratin Infusion Smoothing Conditioner.

STYLERS: Add va-va-voom with a thickening lotion or mousse. Living Proof Full Thickening Cream contains a volumizing molecule called Poly Beta Amino Ester-1, ideal for hair that's not fine. Apply to damp hair from roots to ends. For a sleek look, run a smoothing gel or cream containing phenyl trimethicone, such as Tresemmé Liquid Gold Shine Therapy, through damp hair.

MEDIUM AND DAMAGED

Your strands are thick enough that any hairstyle works, but not so thick that they're tough to manage. The problem? Overstyling (or coloring) has caused split ends, frizz, and dullness. Strengthen with protein and you'll prevent breakage.

SHAMPOO AND CONDITIONER: If hair damage is the result of too much heat styling, hydrolyzed elastin increases flexibility and ceramides or hyaluronic acid moisturize. Tag-team your tresses with Nexus ProMend Daily Shampoo and Conditioner. If you're a bleach-a-holic or are obsessed with chemical straightening, look for fortifying protein or keratin-packed duos, such as Ojon Damage Reverse Restorative Shampoo and Conditioner. If you have both types of damage, alternate the above combos each time you wash.

ONCE A WEEK, coat your hair from midshaft to the ends with an elastin- and fatty acid–rich mask; they provide stress relief and flexibility. Try Wen Sweet Almond Mint Re Moist Intensive Hair Treatment. Postshower, rub in a lightweight leave-in conditioner that contains dimethicone. "It will flatten rough cuticles and reduce frizz," says Thomas.

STYLERS: With all products, remember this: "The damaged regions of hair tend to be negatively charged," says Thomas. "Positively charged ingredients like polyquaterniums, amodimethicone, and bis-aminopropyl dimethicone reinforce weakened hair and prevent heat damage." To play up waves, work an alcohol-free gel, such as L'Oréal Paris EverStyle Curl Defining Gel, into damp hair. Do one small section at a time, gently twisting as you go. Air-dry or use a diffuser. To straighten, work a cream through damp hair. Try John Frieda Frizz Ease Straight Fixation Styling Crème. If you blow-dry, use a boar-bristle brush, says Shorter.

THICK AND HEALTHY

There's an irony to fat strands: Their wide diameters make them voluminous and sexy but also potentially coarser, frizzier, and less shiny than their thinner counterparts. Your mission: Condition! Hydrated thick hair is easier to style and is less poufy.

SHAMPOO: Try to wash only once every 3 days—retaining your hair's natural oils makes it lie better. A cocoa butter–derived cleanser will lock in moisture, making hair softer and shinier. Or pick one that contains shea butter or meadowfoam seed oil, both of which are rich in fuzz-taming fatty acids. Try Fresh Meadowfoam Cream Conditioner.

CONDITIONER: Curly or straight, your hair just loves to tangle. An opaque, buttercream-thick conditioner with behentrimonium chloride or stearalkonium chloride adds slip, meaning you'll be able to remove knots without ripping. Your perfect product: Pantene Pro-V Expert Collection AgeDefy Conditioner.

STYLERS: Avoid products with water as the first ingredient, but don't necessarily skip those that contain alcohol—as long as it's cetyl alcohol, cetearyl alcohol, or stearyl alcohol. These are all fatty acids, which are excellent emollients. Looking to hold shine and eliminate frizz? If your hair isn't coarse, use an oil-based serum (with argan or kernel oil), such as Matrix Biolage Exquisite Oil. If your locks are coarse, go the silicone route with a product like Aussie Smoothing Serum. Make sure the serum is distributed evenly so there aren't spots of greasiness. Shorter recommends separating wet hair into four sections (two on top, two on the bottom). Start with a small amount for your whole head, and divide that into four; rake through each section from roots to tips. If you're straightening with a blow-dryer, use a boar-bristle brush to tame strands delicately.

THICK AND DAMAGED

Your hair is hard to control as it is, but throw in lots of blow-drying, flat-ironing, dyeing, or straightening, and no wonder it's disobeying like a petulant child. Coddle it with mega moisturizers and frizz fighters, and try to use heat tools sparingly.

SHAMPOO: Cleansers with lots of lather—a sign that the detergent level is high—will dehydrate your hair. Safe and nonstripping formulas contain alkyl polyglucosides. You should also look for cuticle-penetrating oils like wheat germ, avocado, and Mombasa oils. Try Clear Scalp and Hair Beauty Therapy Ultra Shea Cleanse and Nourish Shampoo.

CONDITIONER: Give your hair a drink with hydrating power-houses dimethicone, behentrimonium chloride, and stearalkonium chloride. A solid pick: Dove Damage Therapy Intensive Repair Daily Treatment Conditioner. Twice a week, cover dry hair in a deep conditioner with dimethicone or behentrimonium methosulfate. Try Jessicurl Deep Conditioning Treatment.

STYLERS: If you insist on heat styling, first coat towel-dried hair with a serum that has hydrolyzed silk protein or macadamia oil, such as Carol's Daughter Macadamia Heat Protection Serum. For a straight look, try creams or thick oils with silicone and dimethicone—for example, Suave Professionals Moroccan Infusion Moroccan Argan Styling Oil. To enhance waves, mix a nickel-size blob of an alcohol-free curl gel, a silicone-based serum, and a leave-in conditioner in your hand; apply the mixture to damp hair, one small section at a time, gently twisting as you go. Try Tresemmé Mega Firm Control Gel, Mixed Chicks Leave-In Conditioner, and Tigi Catwalk Curl Collection Defining Serum. Air-dry or diffuse your curls. Seal ragged ends with a pomade that has petrolatum or beeswax, such as John Masters Organics Hair Pomade. A final word of caution: Don't try keratin. Layering on too many strengtheners can eliminate damaged hair's ability to be elastic and flexible.

THREE TAKEAWAYS TO TRY TODAY

1. **Layer long hair** to awaken your face and add youthful body.

2. **Add lightweight hydration without dragging down your strands** by using a conditioner containing cetrimonium chloride, cyclomethicone, and glycerin.

3. **Go for foams that don't contain beeswax or candelilla wax.** Waxy styling gels and creams will leave your hair looking flatter than a MacBook Air.

ACKNOWLEDGMENTS

Just as achieving optimal wellness requires tapping different disciplines, philosophies, and practitioners, writing this book was a team effort.

First and foremost, I'd like to thank Laura Tedesco for conducting such remarkable research. Her tireless drive to unearth the most valuable weight-loss, nutrition, and fitness science (and to help translate that into actionable advice) is the foundation on which *20 Pounds Younger* is built.

I am deeply indebted to the doctors, psychologists, nutritionists, trainers, exercise physiologists, and other experts who over the years have carved time out of their busy schedules to impart their wisdom to me. And thanks especially to the awesome group of advisors I call my Life Stylists: Gabrielle Bernstein, Kathryn Budig, Francesca Fusco, Keri Glassman, Holly Perkins, Keri Peterson, Lauren Roxburgh, and Alisa Vitti. I would like to add a shout-out to fitness guru Natalie Uhling, who demonstrated the moves in the training plan with technical precision and inspiring strength. Another indispensible contributor: Jean Kristeller, PhD, professor emeritus of psychology at Indiana State University, who crafted the brilliant 20 Pounds Younger mindful-eating workshop.

I could never have accomplished writing this book without tremendous support from the many talented people at Rodale Books: Thanks to Publisher Mary Ann Naples for her enthusiasm for this project; Marketing Director Brent Gallenberger; Designers Kara Plikaitis and Joanna Williams; Creative Director Jeff Batzli; Managing Editors Chris Krogermeier and Sara Cox; Project Editor Erin Williams; and Editorial Assistant Gillian Francella.

My editor, Jeff Csatari, deserves special recognition. He is a terrific health journalist in his own right and shepherded this book with meticulous care. Thanks also to Rodale CEO Maria Rodale for leading an exceptional company dedicated to the betterment of human and environmental health, and to Rodale President Scott Schulman for his continued support, which I greatly appreciate.

It was my privilege for nearly 6 years to work with an extraordinary team at *Women's Health*, including Publisher Laura Frerer-Schmidt and Director of Communications Lindsey Benoit. And it is now an honor to work with the visionaries at Yahoo Health, in particular Yahoo CMO Kathy Savitt, Rob Barrett, Susan Kittenplan, Jennifer Olsen, Lori Bongiorno, and Becky Auslander.

Above all, I am most grateful to and admiring of readers who actively embrace taking control of their own well-being. Never stop seeking that power.

—MP

Thank you, first and foremost, to the doctors, researchers, and other knowledgeable people who made themselves endlessly available to me. I want to extend a special thanks to Jean Kristeller, PhD, professor emeritus of psychology at Indiana State University, who tirelessly helped me craft the mindful eating workshop that fills the book's final pages, as well as to the Life Stylists who so willingly shared their expertise. And, of course, I'm grateful for my champion and devoted husband, Frank, who kept me energized with caffeine and encouragement during the months spent writing this book.

—LT

Your Mindful Eating Workshop

A Meditation Sequence with Cheese and **Chocolate!**

UNDERSTANDING THE CONCEPT OF MINDFULNESS IS ONE thing—applying it is a whole new experience. Just as you can't wish yourself skinny overnight, you can't miraculously become mindful with a snap of your fingers. Learning to be attentive to your internal experience, thoughts, and bodily sensations takes commitment and practice, which is made infinitely easier by following the schedule on these pages.

This workshop is divided into 6 weeks, plus 1 week of follow-up after you've completed the program. You'll be asked to do a few mindfulness

ABOUT THE EXPERT, JEAN KRISTELLER, PhD

A pioneer of the mindful eating movement, Jean Kristeller, PhD, cofounded the Center for Mindful Eating (thecenterformindfuleating.org) and began developing her renowned Mindfulness-Based Eating Awareness Training (MB-EAT) program over 15 years ago. She is a professor emeritus of psychology at Indiana State University, where she conducts research on meditation, binge eating disorder, and health psychology. The exercises in this workshop are adapted from her MB-EAT programs, developed with the help of Ruth Wolever, PhD, of Duke University.

exercises each week, including one designed to help you become less critical and more accepting of your body. Take at least a day off between meditation and eating exercises so you have time to fully explore your experiences, but continue your writing exercises every day. The point is to do these exercises in an intentional, thoughtful way, without drifting into autopilot mode. Otherwise, they can just become mechanical, which is the exact opposite of being mindful.

Week 1

DAY 1: THE RAISIN MEDITATION

This exercise will teach you to rest your mind only on the present moment and to treat food like a connoisseur does. If you're thirsty, have a glass of water before you begin; you want to avoid drinking during the exercise.

1. Place four raisins on a napkin in front of you, then close your eyes or simply let your gaze fall to the floor in front of you. Take five or six relaxed breaths, noticing the flow of air in and out of your body, the coolness at the tip of your nose as you inhale, followed by the warmth of the air as you exhale. Observe the rising and falling of your stomach and chest with each breath.

2. Open your eyes. Pick up one raisin, examining it as if you've never seen a raisin before, taking note of its wrinkles and color. Now close your eyes, smell the raisin, and then place it against the outside of your lips. What thoughts are popping up in your head? Do you like or dislike raisins? With your eyes still closed, place it in

your mouth without chewing it. Notice how it feels in your mouth, then move it around in your mouth and pay attention to any sensations that crop up.

3. Slowly start to chew the raisin, and experience the taste of just one raisin. Questions to consider: Does it change as you bite into it? What's the flavor like? Where in your mouth are you chewing it? Make sure to notice any thoughts or feelings you have about the raisin.

4. As you prepare to swallow, notice your body's impulse to do so: How does that feel? When you're ready, go ahead and swallow, observing any tastes, sensations, or reactions in your body or mouth. Acknowledge that your body has taken in the weight and energy of one raisin.

5. Now repeat steps 2 through 4, checking for any differences from or similarities to the first raisin. But this time, when you swallow, notice the point at which you can no longer feel the raisin traveling down your throat.

6. Repeat steps 2 through 4 with the third raisin. When you've finished with this one, ask yourself: What am I aware of? Has my body experienced any changes?

7. Now look at the fourth raisin. It's up to you whether or not you eat this one; take a moment to notice your decision-making process. If you decide to eat the raisin, complete the same exercises as you did with the previous raisins.

8. Finally, consider how this raisin came to you—where it may have been planted and grown, how it was dried, how it was delivered to the store where you purchased it. Acknowledge and appreciate the people who helped produce it. Then gently shift your focus back to your breath for two or three breaths, and when you're ready, open your eyes.

REFLECTION

There is no "right" response to eating a raisin. Here are a few questions to help you evaluate your experience.

1. Were you amazed by the flavor intensity of such a small bite?

2. Did you notice subtle differences between the individual raisins?

3. Do you feel surprisingly satisfied after eating just those three or four raisins?

4. Did you think you didn't like raisins but found that you enjoyed them? Or did you think you liked raisins and now realize you don't?

5. What kinds of thoughts or emotions came into your mind?

6. Were there any surprises?

DAY 2: PRACTICING MINDFULNESS MEDITATION

Sometimes meditating is perceived to be just dumping out the contents of your mind, but this isn't accurate: A consistent practice teaches you to observe—and be sensitive to—exactly what's happening in both your mind and body. This can help you control your automatic reactions to experiences—for example, saying "yes" whenever you're offered dessert, regardless of how full you are.

You may find it relaxing to meditate, but you're not trying to make your mind go blank. Rather, you're tuning in to your patterns of thinking and reacting. This can translate to a more pleasurable eating experience while helping you connect with your "inner wisdom"—the ability to listen to your body's signals. Developing inner wisdom is the key to weight loss because you'll learn to identify when you're truly physically hungry (rather than emotionally hungry) and when you've eaten enough. You'll also be able to recognize your emotions and thoughts about food without reacting to them automatically.

Repetition is key: The more you practice meditation, the easier you'll find it is to manage your eating—and that is related to greater weight loss and improved mood. Realizing that your practice is individual is just as important: You may catch on quickly, or it may take you weeks to get the hang of it. That's okay, as long as you stick with it.

INTRODUCTION TO MINDFULNESS MEDITATION

> Sit in a chair or on the floor with a relaxed but erect posture that you can easily maintain, and rest your hands in your lap. Setting a timer for 10 or 15 minutes, possibly in another room, is recommended.

> Close your eyes, then sit completely still. Start by taking three or four deep breaths from your diaphragm, letting the air flow fully into your stomach, without any pushing, and then gently flow back out again. Notice your increasing sense of calm as you progress through your breaths.

> Allow your breathing to fall into a natural, comfortable rhythm and depth. How does your breath feel as it enters at the tip of your nose, moves through the back of your throat, into your lower diaphragm, and then back out again? Is the air cooler coming in, then warmer on its way out? Determine the point in your breath that you find easiest to focus on.

> Thoughts and feelings *will* crop up: You may find yourself obsessing over a certain bodily sensation or noise, thinking about the past, or getting lost in fantasy. You just have to return your attention to your breath—without any self-judgment. Can't quite cut out the internal criticism? Label it as such—*I'm judging myself for my wandering mind*—and choose to move on. Remember, you can briefly acknowledge the concerns or feelings that distract you as long as you let go of them just as quickly.

> If returning to your breathing isn't enough to take your mind off your thoughts, imagine your mental chatter drifting by, like clouds blown by a breeze. Or, if that doesn't work, you can count from 1 to 10 with each breath for a few minutes to help you become more focused. Don't try to push away your thoughts—becoming aware of them, then shifting your focus to your breathing, is more important than trying to silence them.

> Likewise, if you become preoccupied by emotions—anxiety, sadness, anger, frustration with your body—simply allow them to pass through, without being drawn in or engaging in the train of thought that follows. Notice how the feeling shifts or changes, while acknowledging that thoughts are just thoughts, and then return to your breath.

> If it's a physical sensation (such as restlessness) that's disturbing your practice, you can choose to move slightly, while noticing how that

movement feels and focusing on the point of discomfort as if you're watching it from afar (rather than actively feeling it). Notice the word "choose"—this isn't automatically stirring because you're uncomfortable. Rather, you're deciding that you will consciously alter your body position.

> Shift your focus back to your breath, and when the timer sounds, begin to gently move around in your chair. When you're ready, open your eyes and stretch out.

REFLECTION

Do you feel . . .

1.   *Relaxed and comfortable?* Consider your first session a success!

2.   *Plagued by intrusive, troublesome thoughts?* If you experienced highly uncomfortable feelings during your practice, try shortening your meditation sessions and keeping your eyes partially open, with a half-focused gaze on the floor in front of you.

3.   *Like a failure, because you couldn't stay focused?* A racing mind doesn't mean you were meditating incorrectly. It's a sign of progress that you were even aware of your mental chatter! No matter your level of experience, thoughts and feelings will crop up. You just have to notice them, let them go, and return to your breath without beating yourself up. Think of them as birds flying through the sky of your mind: You can notice them without following them.

4.   *Ready to drift off?* If you felt on the brink of sleep, you may need to rely less on your chair's backrest and more on your spine to maintain upright posture. Or change your practice time to when you're better rested.

APPLICATION

Aim to practice mindfulness meditation every day. To ease into a routine, start with just 10 minutes of daily practice (or less, if that feels daunting), and gradually progress to 20 minutes once (or twice) a day. As you figure out how to fit this into your schedule, try to anticipate any potential distractions—such as a yappy dog or young children—and figure out ways to work around them. This may require asking family members not to disturb you, possibly even setting a timer for them in a different room, and experimenting with different times and places to practice. The ultimate goal is to establish a consistent meditation schedule.

If you commit to regular practice, you'll start to reap long-term rewards: greater awareness, relaxation, and control over your life when you really need it: throughout the day and when you're eating. You can still learn to meditate if you skip a day or two, but your progress will be slower and less profound.

Week 2

DAY 1: INTRODUCTION TO MINI MEDITATIONS

The formal, sitting style of meditation you've already learned teaches you to cultivate your overall capacity for mindfulness and helps you apply the skill in a wide range of daily situations. Short, mini meditations just before eating can help you bring mindfulness to the table. Just pause for a few brief moments; take a few deep breaths; tune in to your thoughts, feelings, and level of hunger; and stamp out mindless eating before it starts.

1. Your first mini meditation should be done at home, when you're eating alone. Place your feet flat on the floor, rest your hands comfortably in your lap, and close your eyes. Take several deep, relaxing breaths into your stomach (not your chest). Notice if any areas of your body feel tense, and if so, imagine that you're breathing specifically into those areas, releasing any tension or discomfort.

2. Keeping your eyes closed, picture the food in front of you. Inhale slowly, then exhale, once again focusing on any tension in your body. Notice, without judgment, any feelings or thoughts about the food in front of you or experiences that are distracting you, especially those that are related to the food or a desire to eat right now.

3. Continue breathing in and out, bringing awareness to any tension in your body. Take one more deep breath, and open your eyes when you're ready.

REFLECTION

How might mini meditations help you bring a more balanced approach to eating?

APPLICATION

Perform a brief mini meditation before at least one meal or snack per day, working up to every time you eat. If you find yourself forgetting to do so, try placing a sticker on your fridge or pantry to remind yourself. You can also use mini meditations briefly during meals, and with practice, you'll find that you can bring yourself into this brief moment of mindful awareness more and more easily, without closing your eyes or needing to take breaths to relax.

DAY 2: MINDFULLY EATING CHEESE AND CRACKERS

Now it's time to increase the challenge by mindfully eating cheese and crackers, a higher-fat snack that is much easier to eat in excess than raisins. We're not asking you to give up any one food entirely, but rather to learn to appreciate and truly enjoy smaller amounts of "less healthy" ones. (This is unlike traditional diet programs, which usually deal with high-fat foods by cutting them out completely.) A flexible approach means you'll inevitably face foods that you've consistently overeaten in the past, so you have to learn how to eat them in a more balanced manner.

1. If possible, use a presliced, high-quality, mild cheddar cheese paired with small crackers, such as Wheat Thins. Cutting a sandwich-size slice of cheese like a tic-tac-toe board produces small squares that fit perfectly on a Wheat Thin. Or you can use a larger cracker, like saltines, and cut the cheese into four pieces. Allow the cheese to reach room temperature (it's more flavorful when slightly warm), and place three or four cheese-and-cracker pairs on a plate in front of you.

2. Close your eyes and take several deep, relaxing breaths. Are any parts of your body tense? If so, breathe into these areas, and let go of the tension. Without criticizing yourself, observe any feelings, experiences, or thoughts cropping up in your mind, particularly those related to the food in front of you. Breathe in again, and open your eyes.

3. Pick up one cracker topped with cheese, and examine it as if you're a food connoisseur. Take a moment to smell it, then close your eyes and either place the whole thing in your mouth or take a bite of it. Before you begin chewing, move it around in your mouth. What sensations are you experiencing?

4. As you start to chew, notice how the taste changes. Savor the experience of eating this small piece of food, and observe the satisfaction you get from it. Notice how your body, thoughts, emotions, and mind react to the food. Try to take about a minute to do this.

5. Choose to swallow. Pay attention to how you feel once the cheese and cracker are gone: Are any sensations still lingering in your mouth?

6. Open your eyes just enough so you can see and take a second cracker. Look at it, close your eyes, smell it, and place it in your mouth, experiencing the taste and texture before chewing it.

7. Once you begin chewing, notice how each cracker or bite of cracker may differ from the previous one. Draw as much satisfaction and pleasure as possible from each bite, and notice any thoughts or feelings, without judgment, as they arise.

8. Once again, choose to swallow, and notice the experience of doing so, as you shift your mental focus to your breath.

9. Does your body or mind want another cracker? If so, help yourself to the next one, and lead yourself through eating it mindfully. If you don't want the last cracker, return your awareness to your breath. Whether you're eating or not, pay attention to any thoughts and feelings that arise. Reflect on all the steps that made this little snack come into being—that brought it here to nourish you. If you're eating, decide to swallow, and take a moment to appreciate the fuel you're providing to your body.

10. Bring your awareness back to your breath, your body, and then the room. When you're ready, open your eyes.

REFLECTION

> What was it like eating food this way? How did mindfully eating a high-fat food differ from eating the raisins mindfully?

> What did you notice about your thoughts and feelings?

> How could you apply this exercise to other foods at home? At social events? How would this differ from your usual approach to eating?

> If you found yourself feeling nervous about the calories or fat in this snack, you might check the cheese package and cracker box to see how much "food energy" you actually took in. (Most people are actually surprised by how few calories they consumed!)

> Keep in mind that eating mindfully doesn't always mean eating this slowly. As you become more aware, you'll find that you can maintain a mindful perspective while eating at a more normal pace.

APPLICATION

Aim to eat at least one meal mindfully each day. If you want to apply your new skills to more meals, go for it!

DAY 3: LONGER MEDITATION PRACTICE

Congratulations, you've now been meditating for almost a week! That's more than most people have ever done. This exercise is designed to help you advance toward your goal of 20-minute meditation sessions. During this meditation, you want to work on "noting"—that is, briefly labeling whatever comes into your awareness, using words such as "noise," "itch," "worry thought," or "planning thought." This can help you establish a more objective awareness, quelling the desire to react automatically to every experience. Don't worry too much about accurately labeling your experience; the goal is just to interrupt your usual reactivity to or awareness of an experience.

Restlessness and boredom count as feelings, so take note when these arise by briefly and silently labeling them. If you find yourself sinking into self-criticism, simply shift your focus to your breathing or mantra.

Refer to last week's "Introduction to Mindfulness Meditation" for instructions (see page 227), this time setting your timer for 20 minutes.

REFLECTION

> How is your daily meditation practice going? Do you find it easier to meditate the more you practice?

> Is your mental awareness of your thoughts and feelings improving?

> Are you becoming more aware of your chattering mind, thoughts, and feelings—both while meditating and at other times of the day? Are you just observing them, rather than reacting to them?

Week 3

DAY 1: CHECK-IN

By now, you've probably seen some positive shifts in your eating. Hopefully you feel more balanced—realizing you can enjoy eating smaller amounts of food without feeling a constant yearning to eat more and more. Even if you've reverted to old eating habits on occasion, you've still laid the groundwork to overcome them down the road just by mindfully eating one meal a day. So good job, you're making progress!

OVER THE LAST FEW DAYS ...

Have you noticed any changes in your eating experiences as a result of last week's cheese-and-crackers exercise?

_____

_____

_____

_____

_____

Have you been doing mini meditations before meals or snacks? During meals or snacks? How have they helped you be more mindful?

_____

_____

_____

_____

_____

Have you slipped back into the old habit of getting mad at yourself when you mess up, rather than being curious about why it happened? How do you handle it if this happens?

_____

_____

_____

_____

_____

DAY 2: INTRODUCTION OF HUNGER AWARENESS

A core component of mindful eating is learning to tune in to physical hunger signals from your body, then gradually starting to distinguish these cues from other eating triggers, whether emotional, environmental, or social. The key to using meditation to curb overeating is cultivating the inner wisdom that comes from listening to your body's hunger signals (not just trying to ignore them). This concept may seem totally foreign to you, since many diet programs only try to suppress or evade your hunger, rather than deal with it. With a little practice and a lot of attention, your discernment will develop over time.

To hone your internal intuition, you also have to pinpoint the challenges that meddle with your body's signals, such as boredom and anxiety, both of which can trick you into thinking you're hungry. You may be tempted to order a margarita and a basket of wings to celebrate, to eat a pint of ice cream after a day from hell, or to have a second or third slice of pizza just because your super-in-shape gal pal is. We all fall victim to this kind of thinking. But instead of kicking yourself later and thinking you're a failure, acknowledge these urges as they occur, then decide to make a choice that aligns with how your body really feels. It gets a little easier every time.

First, a few questions to consider:

> What does physical hunger mean?

> How is it different from psychological hunger?

> Do you feel afraid of being at all hungry? If yes, why?

Working with a hunger scale can help you objectively assess your need to feed and tune out the emotions that often override your body's signals. Do this exercise, ideally checking in before your usual meal times and then several hours after a meal.

1.   Sit in a chair with your spine straight and your feet flat on the floor. Bring your attention to your breath, closing your eyes if you wish.

2. Follow your breath as you inhale and exhale a few times, then determine how physically hungry you are, with 10 being as hungry as possible and 0 being not hungry at all. There is no right or wrong answer.

3. Once you've decided upon your number, ask yourself: What sensations or experiences helped me determine this number?

4. Return your focus to your breathing, then back to the room. When you're ready, open your eyes.

Repeating this exercise at different times of day—before a meal, 2 hours after eating, 5 hours after eating—will help you establish your own personal hunger scale.

Not at all hungry				Moderately hungry					Very hungry	
0	1	2	3	4	5	6	7	8	9	10

REFLECTION

> Think about times when you've been very hungry. What did that feel like?

> Now, if very hungry feels the way you've described it, what does moderately hungry feel like? A little hungry?

APPLICATION

Chances are, you found the last question more difficult to answer than the first. That's normal. During the week, try to track the sensations associated with moderate hunger, and notice your hunger levels throughout the day and around each snack or meal. Keep in mind that you shouldn't wait until you're famished—a 9 or 10 on your hunger scale—to eat, since this may contribute to overeating. Note: You don't have to always use the numbers on the scale, but it's very helpful to get an idea of some of the meaningful differences in hunger experiences for yourself.

DAY 3: INTRODUCTION TO EMOTIONAL EATING AND OTHER TRIGGERS

True physical hunger is not the only reason most of us eat. The primary focus of this exercise is emotional eating, but you should realize that there are many other external triggers for chowing down, including the mere presence of appetizing food, social occasions, and long-standing habits of eating during certain activities (such as watching TV).

It's important to note that most people—regardless of their weight—are more likely to eat in response to emotions and other external cues. Some folks just fall prey to emotional eating less frequently than others, compensate by eating less later in the day, or pick foods with higher nutritional value when they do eat for these reasons.

It's not necessarily bad or wrong to eat for a reason other than hunger. But if it's out of control and you're not even aware that you do it, this type of eating can contribute to major weight gain, especially if food is your primary way to cope with stress.

Fill in this chart to help you identify the non-hunger-related signals that compel you to munch.

POSITIVE EMOTIONS THAT DRIVE ME TO EAT	NEGATIVE EMOTIONS THAT DRIVE ME TO EAT	NONEMOTIONAL TRIGGERS THAT DRIVE ME TO EAT

If you realize that you sometimes eat because of emotions, how do you distinguish between physical and emotional hunger? Are there any different signals you're aware of?

_____

_____

_____

_____

_____

The more you pay attention to your mindset when you start munching—use those mini meditations!—the better you'll become at recognizing the things that drive your eating. ("Am I eating because I'm angry? Bored? Anxious? Or perhaps I'm just procrastinating?") Sometimes emotions are subtle—you don't necessarily have to be boiling mad or crazy stressed to crave a box of doughnuts. And yes, you *can* be physically hungry and emotionally hungry at the same time, which adds an extra layer of confusion to this whole process—but also means that you might want to eat something particularly satisfying.

Some themes you may notice as you delve into your emotional life may include self-soothing (you had a stressful day, so you deserve ice cream), entertainment (you have nothing better to do), rebellion (you swore you wouldn't eat chocolate, but screw that, you're having some!), or control (you feel out of control in your life, but nobody can tell you how to eat).

REFLECTION

Which foods do you typically eat for emotional reasons? List them below along with the related emotions.

_____

_____

_____

_____

_____

APPLICATION

If you're keeping a food log, which can be helpful when you're getting used to a new way of eating, make a special effort to jot down your emotions before each meal or snack. After several days, look back over your entries, and see if any emotional-eating trends emerge, such as grabbing a latte whenever you're stressed or eating ice cream when you're sad.

DAY 4: BODY SCAN

If you've ever struggled with your weight, you probably have some pretty negative feelings attached to food. But the food itself may not be the root of the issue; problematic eating may boil down to a lack of body acceptance. If your weight is a source of stress, you may have long ago shut off your mind's awareness of your body out of fear, anxiety, or distress over how you think your body looks. This can make it tough to read your body's signals, since the capacity to understand (and accept) your needs starts with comfort in your own skin.

The following exercise is designed to instill a sense of self-care—a way of loving your body, taking care of it, and being kind to it that doesn't involve food.

1. Spend a moment relaxing in any way that's comfortable to you. Just let go—allow your body to be loose and at ease. Relax each part of your body—your feet, your legs, your stomach, your shoulders, your arms, your neck, and your face.

2. Now bring awareness to your body, to some specific place. Where does your attention go? Notice any thoughts and feelings about that body part, whether positive or negative.

3. Focus your feeling on the center of your body. How comfortable are you allowing your attention to be focused on your body? Just notice, without judging.

4. As you stay relaxed, briefly scan your body and determine if there is any place that particularly grabs your attention. Rest your mind there as if you are intently listening to what your body might say.

5. Still staying relaxed, rest your awareness on a place in your body that creates some feelings of discomfort. Be aware of the discomfort. If the feelings are too intense, move to another area where the discomfort is less disturbing. Stay with that discomfort, without judging or analyzing it. Just let those feelings rise and fall.

6. Now shift your focus back to your breath, let yourself relax, and let go of any lingering feelings. Remain relaxed, then briefly scan your body one more time, noticing a place that calls your attention in a positive way—a body part that you're proud of. Acknowledge the incredible work your feet, wrists, lungs, and heart do for you. Appreciate how awesome your body is in helping you live your life. Return your attention again to some body part you're proud of, without analyzing it.

7. Bring your attention back to your breath. Thank your body for any communication or new awareness you achieved.

REFLECTION

> What was the most difficult part of this exercise?

> What was useful about it? What did you discover?

> What thoughts or feelings cropped up during this exercise?

> What's the difference between self-acceptance and self-judgment? Between self-acceptance and not caring?

> In the past, did you think that judging yourself was necessary for change?

APPLICATION

Continue your daily meditation practice (now ideally 20 minutes long), which you can end with a brief body scan, and do mini meditations before and during meals or snacks. Eat at least one or two meals mindfully every day, paying special attention to your level of physical hunger before and during the meal and the nature of physical hunger versus other cues for eating.

Your new challenge: Try to eat only when you're physically hungry, rather than according to the clock or just because food is available. Experiment with this throughout the day. You may find it easiest, for example, to eat exclusively for hunger in the morning or at lunchtime. As part of this task, start paying attention to your level of emotional hunger and other eating triggers, along with your physical hunger, and bring more focus to your body during the week.

Week 4

DAY 1: CHECK-IN

You've completed 3 weeks of mindful eating. Give yourself a pat on the back! Is it starting to feel like second nature, or are you still struggling to get used to it? Briefly jot down any positive or challenging experiences from the previous week, including your experiences with paying attention to physical versus emotional hunger cues, choosing to eat only when physically hungry, and noticing the strength of eating triggers when you're less physically hungry. Remember, your eating patterns have developed over many years, and it will take more than a few weeks to develop a new relationship with eating and food.

_____

_____

_____

_____

Have you been able to eat one or two meals mindfully each day? Have you been doing mini meditations before and during snacks and meals? Write down any struggles or successes.

_____

_____

_____

_____

_____

DAY 2: TASTE SATISFACTION—MINDFULLY EATING CHOCOLATE

So far, we've focused on recognizing when you're physically hungry and when to *start* eating. Now we're addressing the second half of that equation: when to *stop* eating—which many people do only when their plate is empty. You may have heard that it takes 20 minutes before your body tells you to stop. You can eat a lot of food in 20 minutes! Think about your own "stop eating" signals. Are these internal or external cues? Is it something inside or outside your body that tells you to set down the fork? The good news is that these internal signals kick in much sooner than 20 minutes.

The first signal to tune into: taste satiety. The last bite of a meal is never as good as the first because your palate stops responding as strongly to the taste of food over the course of a meal. You may find it helpful to think of taste satiety—and the related concept of taste satisfaction from 1 to 10— much in the same way that you think about hunger, but on a meter that can move up and down rather than on a simple scale. How high the meter shoots up is related to how much you like the food, but your taste buds getting tired causes the satisfaction meter to drop, regardless of how high it starts. Think back to the cheese-and-crackers task: How quickly did your taste perception shift from "good" or even "amazing" to "I've had enough"? You may have even noticed this with the raisins. Now you're going to try it with chocolate!

The point of this exercise isn't just to indulge—it's to teach you about taste satisfaction and taste satiety. Taste satisfaction is how much you enjoy a food. Your level of pleasure will be higher for foods you really like or those that are higher quality. Taste satiety is the reduction of taste satisfaction as your taste buds start to get tired, regardless of the initial level of satisfaction. Eating more and more to regain the pleasure of the first couple of bites is futile—"chasing the flavor" simply doesn't reawaken your senses. Can this really happen with something as enticing as chocolate?

Most of us resort to "problem" foods to meet nonphysical needs: We down a giant bag of candy when we're stressed, a bag of chips when we're bored, or a heaping bowl of ice cream after a breakup. Since these are the foods we're often most drawn to in times of trouble (or even celebration), it's important to learn how to eat them in moderation, with maximum pleasure.

1. Cut up a few chocolate cookies and/or brownies into small wedges or 1-inch squares. Choose a brand that seems appealing, that you'd buy or choose as a snack, but not necessarily the highest quality possible. As you cultivate your inner gourmand, you can work up to that kind! Place the cookies or brownies on a plate, paying attention to the appearance of the items as you arrange them.

2. Close your eyes and take several deep, relaxing breaths. Notice your level of hunger: On a scale of 1 to 10, what is it? How do you know that?

3. Now open your eyes, and look at the plate in front of you. Pick up one piece and look at it carefully, as if you're seeing this food for the first time.

4. Close your eyes again, and bring the chocolate to your nose and smell it. Place it into your mouth without biting it. Just notice how it feels in your mouth. Then as you bite into it, notice how the taste changes, and where your taste satisfaction meter is, with 10 being as satisfying as possible and 1 being not satisfying at all. Allow yourself to enjoy this small piece of food as fully as possible, and observe how your body is reacting. How does your body feel? Is your taste satisfaction changing? Maybe it goes up, down, or stays the same.

5. Decide to swallow, and pay attention to the experience—how your body responds, the flavors that are still in your mouth, the thoughts and emotions you're having.

6. With your eyes still closed, take several deep, relaxing breaths, and notice your level of hunger: Is it the same? Has it changed? How do you know this?

7. Open your eyes just enough to pick up a second chocolate piece. Examine it carefully, noticing any thoughts or feelings, then close your eyes again and smell the chocolate. Place it in your mouth

without biting it, and determine if it feels any different than the first piece.

8. As you bite into it, notice any changes in the taste or other sensations from the first piece as you slowly savor it. Where is your taste satisfaction meter this time? How is your body reacting?

9. Choose to swallow, being aware of the point at which you lose the sensation of food in your throat. Notice any lingering flavors in your mouth and whether you feel hungry.

10. Now take a third piece of chocolate, and lead yourself through the experience of eating it mindfully, noticing the level of taste satisfaction you reach. Does your taste satiety change as you eat?

11. It's your decision whether you eat the fourth piece of chocolate. Either way is fine—just notice how you decide to eat more or to stop, being mindful of the reason behind your choice.

12. Bring awareness back to your breath, then to the room, and when you're ready, slowly open your eyes.

REFLECTION

> What did you notice about your taste satisfaction? Did it change?

> Did anything surprise you?

> What did you notice about how you made the decision to eat more or to stop eating?

> Did your hunger change over the course of the exercise?

> Did you find yourself wanting to eat more chocolate to "chase the flavor"?

Most people find that they feel satisfied with less chocolate than they thought they would be. If you feel differently, keep repeating this exercise on your own. It may simply have been so long since you focused on taste that you need more practice.

APPLICATION

Try this exercise with different foods, in different amounts, and at different levels of hunger.

DAY 3: LEARNING WHEN TO SET THE FORK DOWN

A change in taste satisfaction is usually the first satiety signal to kick in. Next comes the actual feeling of physical fullness, which can range from a little bit of pressure to a bloated belly. Most people can quickly learn to differentiate between low, moderate, and higher levels of fullness, even if they've spent years eating past the point of discomfort. Just as you learned to rate your hunger on a 10-point scale and your taste satisfaction on a 10-point meter, so you'll be scoring your fullness:

Not at all full				Moderately full						Very full
0	1	2	3	4	5	6	7	8	9	10

It's pretty easy to identify when you're not at all or completely full. But how do you know when you're slightly full? One sign: You've eaten a snack or small meal, but you could still easily exercise. Your level of comfort is also a cue: If you're moderately full, you may feel a stretch in your stomach, but you don't have the distended belly that most people refer to as "full." If you learn to spot these signals, you can learn to mindfully choose when to stop eating.

There is no absolutely right level of fullness. At some meals, you might prefer to keep it light, perhaps so you can hit the gym afterward. At a festive family meal, eating to the point of feeling somewhat uncomfortable might seem fine; however, eating that much at most meals doesn't represent a mindful choice, but rather a set of habits or patterns that may be leading to other problems.

It is possible to *feel* physically full without having consumed any (or many) actual nutrients—physical fullness is really just a matter of space in your stomach—whereas the blood sugar response occurs only after you've taken in nutrient-containing food. Your stomach isn't just a mechanical space; it interacts with the quality of your food, which means that your sense of body satiety and fullness may increase after a meal more so with some foods than with others.

The following exercise is designed to help you hone in on the physical sensation of fullness, separate from feelings of body satiety. Plan to do this exercise when you are at least somewhat hungry.

STOMACH FULLNESS MEDITATION (10 MINUTES)

1. Sit with an upright posture, your feet flat on the floor. Place a 16- to 20-ounce bottle of water on a table in front of you. Close your eyes, place your hands on your stomach, and take three or four easy, deep breaths. Don't force your breath—just invite it all the way to the bottom of your lungs. As the air reaches the bottom of your lungs, you may feel your abdomen expand on the inhale and contract on the exhale. Just notice the sensations you're experiencing.

2. On a scale of 1 to 10, how hungry are you right now? What are you feeling in your stomach? On a scale of 1 to 10, how full are you, with 10 being as full as possible and 1 being not full at all? How do you know that? Take a moment to be aware of all of the sensations that are telling you your level of fullness.

3. Now open your eyes, grab your bottle of water, and quickly drink about half of it. Observe any changes in the feelings in your stomach, closing your eyes if you wish. On a scale of 1 to 10, how full are you right now?

4. Again, open your eyes, grab your bottle of water, and drink the rest of it (or as much as you possibly can). Close your eyes if you wish, then rate your fullness, as well as your hunger, on a scale of 1 to 10.

5. Return your attention to your breath, taking a few more deep, relaxing breaths, and then gently open your eyes.

REFLECTION

> How did your level of fullness change over the course of this meditation?

> How would eating this same amount of food differ from drinking this amount of water?

> ❯ What types of situations, emotions, or thoughts might get in the way of recognizing fullness or might be related to eating after you're full?

APPLICATION

Being aware of fullness and deciding whether or not to continue eating are two different things. (We've all been there—totally stuffed, yet still feasting.) Over the next few days, simply try to observe your feelings of fullness and rate them on a 10-point scale at several points in time, such as just before a meal, several times during a meal, just after a meal, an hour after a meal, and 2 hours after a meal.

Week 5

DAY 1: THE RELATIONSHIP BETWEEN HUNGER, FULLNESS, AND BODY SATIETY

You have a lot going on during a meal: Your hunger is decreasing, your fullness is increasing, and your body satiety is gradually kicking in as the food is absorbed. Here's where it gets especially complicated: Hunger and fullness are distinct bodily processes that are controlled by different parts of your brain and body, even though most of us experience them as a single system. In other words, just because hunger is decreasing doesn't mean fullness is increasing (or vice versa). Think about the two rating scales this way:

Most hungry										Least hungry
10	9	8	7	6	5	4	3	2	1	0

0	1	2	3	4	5	6	7	8	9	10
Least full										Most full

It is possible to be quite hungry and (as you did in a previous exercise) drink a large glass of water, experience a sense of physical fullness, and yet still be hungry. It's also possible to eat a small amount of satisfying food, quickly feel less hungry and more satiated as the nutrients are absorbed, but still have your stomach feel relatively empty.

APPLICATION

During meals and snacks this week, observe your increase in physical fullness as meals progress, as well as your feelings of satiety during and after the eating experience. Take note of how stomach fullness may continue to increase after you stop eating, as part of the body satiety process.

DAY 2: HEALING SELF-TOUCH*

It's an unfortunate reality: Few people who are overweight sincerely feel good about their bodies. The healing practice of self-touch, which builds on the body scan exercise, is intended to help you engage with—and then begin to overcome—the feelings of shame, distrust, self-rejection, sadness, or hurt that stem from dissatisfaction with your body. This requires directing your attention to common "trouble" spots—your stomach, your thighs—as well as to other, more neutral areas of your body.

As challenging as it may be to face how you really feel about your figure, this exercise will ultimately help you become more aware of your body, and that can improve your ability to notice your internal hunger signals and emotional motivations for eating. In fact, recent British research suggests that loving self-touch may boost your sense of body ownership, which is key if you want to regain a sense of self-control.

1. Spend a moment finding a comfortable posture. As you relax, take several deep, full breaths, in and out, closing your eyes if you wish.

2. Bring your attention to your hands, noticing the sensation of whatever they are touching. Now imagine your palms are filling up with kindness, caring, warmth, and tenderness.

3. Lift one hand and place it on the opposite arm, touching your skin gently and with care. Notice what this feels like, the sensation of touching. How are you reacting? Focus first on the surface of your arm, then let your attention move deep into its center—to the bones that give your arm strength, to the muscles that allow it to move. What is going through your mind? Notice, without judgment, any thoughts that come up. Gently move your hand up and down your arm with a kind touch, focusing on both the surface and what lies beneath. Now repeat the process with your other hand on the opposite arm.

4. Move both hands, still imagining them being filled with kindness, to your thighs, gently placing them wherever is most comfortable. If you're able, touch your thighs with a sense of appreciation for the bones and muscles that hold you up and allow you to move. Notice any feelings of tenderness this may bring, then gently caress your thighs and further down your legs, if you so choose.

5. Slowly move your hands to your stomach, observing its movement as you breathe. How are you reacting? Continue to imagine your hands being filled with kindness and, while maintaining a sense of tenderness, acknowledge all of the organs that allow you to live.

6. Finally, place one hand over your heart, observing your breathing and your heartbeat, if you can. Feel the compassionate quality of your heart, and allow it to flow through your hands. If mental chatter pops up, let it come and go, returning to a sense of caring and kindness. In these last few moments, if you feel there is another part of your body that could use a caring, tender touch, move your hands there, and rest in a sense of appreciation.

7. Bring your awareness back to your breath, and when you're ready, open your eyes.

---

* The healing self-touch exercise was developed by Sasha Loring, MS, MEd, at Duke Integrative Medicine.

REFLECTION

> ❯ Was this exercise difficult for you? Useful?
> ❯ What feelings or thoughts did you experience?
> ❯ What did you discover?
> ❯ How might this self-touch exercise influence weight loss?
> ❯ Which parts of your body did you find easiest to appreciate? Hardest?

DAY 3: MINDFULLY CHOOSING BETWEEN COOKIES AND CHIPS

Mindless eating can also mean grabbing the first food that's convenient, rather than the one that you really want to eat. If you don't mindfully decide which snack you want, you may not feel the surge in pleasure you hoped for, and you will then continue grazing. So a key part of mindful eating is pausing before you dig in to bring awareness to your food choices, whether it's between two foods or among many. What you're trying to figure out: How do you know when a food is calling to you? How can you mindfully choose the right snack so you avoid eating several different foods without ever feeling satisfied? Do this exercise when you haven't recently eaten.

1. Place a handful of small, rich cookies (such as Lorna Doones) and corn chips (such as Fritos) on a single plate. These two snacks are similar in color and each is uniform in flavor (no nuts or chocolate chips in the cookies, no complex seasonings in the chips).

2. Move into a mindful meditative state, slowing down your breathing. Rate how physically hungry you are on a scale of 1 to 10. How do you know this?

3. Now rate how full you are, again on a scale of 1 to 10. What about your body satiety—where does it fall on a scale of 1 to 10? How do you know this?

4. Take a few minutes to look at the food. Consider which snack you'd prefer at this particular moment—sweet or salty? Reflect on how you made this choice, then take *more* than you think you want to eat of

only this snack and place the plate with the remaining food out of your direct sight. Observe the food you've chosen, noticing its shape and color, wondering where this food came from.

5. Now check in again with your body: Rate your hunger and fullness from 1 to 10. Pick up a piece, smell it, then close your eyes. Bring the food to your lips and feel its texture before biting into it. Once you take a bite, chew slowly, being aware of how and where in your mouth you experience the food and how much you're enjoying it. Notice how high your internal taste meter went after the first bite, on a scale of 1 to 10. With each bite, notice whether it goes up, down, or stays the same. Is it going up as high as you expected? Higher? Continue to eat the rest of the cookie or chip in this way, noticing any changes in flavor and enjoying the taste of the food as much as possible.

6. Stop when you've eaten everything you took or you no longer want any more. Now check in and rate your hunger and fullness, then open your eyes. Bring the plate with the remaining snacks back in front of you. You have a choice: Take more of what you already had, or take a little of the other food. How are you making this decision?

7. Whatever you choose, lead yourself through eating this snack mindfully. If you took the second food, how is it different from the first? If you took more of the first food, are there any surprises? With each bite, rate the pleasure of the taste from 1 to 10 on your taste meter. Notice whether it goes up, goes down, or stays the same. Stop eating when you've eaten everything on your plate or you no longer enjoy the food.

8. Appreciate what it is that you've taken into your body, and rest your hand on your stomach. Be aware of any feelings of hunger or fullness. Notice any judgment you have. Then gently open your eyes.

REFLECTION

> The primary focus of this exercise is tuning in to how to make a choice between two foods, but it also wove together hunger awareness, fullness awareness, taste satiety, satisfaction awareness, and food choices. Which were harder to observe? Which were easier?

> What was surprising about this exercise? What did you find interesting?

> Did you find that you wanted to keep eating?

> Did you notice a change in taste as you ate? On the taste satisfaction meter, how satisfied did you feel with your snack, from 1 to 10? What might contribute to your feelings of satisfaction?

> Did you experience a change in body satiety?

APPLICATION

Repeat this experiment with different foods and levels of hunger. Specifically, try this same exercise with your favorite comfort foods—those you tend to turn to in times of stress or trouble.

DAY 4: BREAKING THE CHAIN OF OVEREATING

Out-of-control eating doesn't come out of nowhere. If you look hard enough, you'll almost always find a trigger. It may be a negative thought, like, "I've already blown it, since I ate one doughnut," or even a positive thought, like, "I deserve this." It could be an emotion—boredom, stress, anger, rejection— or just an activity, such as watching TV, that drives you to eat. This process of examining the factors that drove you to overdo it is called "chain analysis." Think about it like this:

You have a bad day at work » *You start obsessing over your boss's criticism* » *You comfort yourself by ordering a burger-and-fries combo—and opt to supersize it*

Sometimes there are several links in the chain, but the process of figuring out what triggered you to overeat is the same. Work backwards, starting with the eating event: You slurped down a large milk shake in 5 minutes flat. Ask yourself: "What was I thinking right before I started eating?" Fill in the previous link on the chain. Then consider what happened right before that, and fill in the next link. Continue until you've created a chain of thoughts, feelings, sensations, or behaviors—some intense, others relatively mundane—that lead you to the underlying causes of your overeating.

As you work through this process, carefully distinguish between thoughts and emotions. Your thought might be, "My boss will never appreciate me," while the underlying emotion is frustration. For every thought there's probably an emotion, and vice versa. Try to identify both. If you find yourself dwelling on outside circumstances—for example, the cookies were practically staring you down—return to your reaction: What happened inside you when you saw those cookies?

Being mindful is not always easy. It often requires sitting and observing difficult emotions, thoughts, or cravings, or doing what's called "surfing the urge." The goal is to ride out the wave, rather than getting swept away—and finding yourself face-first in a bag of tortilla chips. But remember, even if you start overeating, you can interrupt that process at any point; two cookies always have fewer calories than four—and might leave you feeling satisfied, rather than guilty.

This meditation is designed to help you do this from a nonjudgmental and compassionate perspective—and to help you realize how much choice you really have when it comes to eating.

> ❭ Close your eyes and sit with an easy, straight posture. Find a position that allows gravity to gently maintain your proper posture. Rest your hands in your lap.

> ❭ Focus on your breath, so your mind shifts away from the noise—the thoughts, concerns, or feelings that usually fill your mind. Now imagine yourself during a typical day. This day is like any other, but for one difference: You will overeat. Try to remain detached, as an objective observer, as you watch the events leading up to the overeating incident unfold. Don't picture yourself eating compulsively—just notice what happened before you ate, in the time leading up to it, and perhaps before you realized you would overeat. What took place? What time was it? Notice your surroundings: Are you alone or with others?

> ❭ Now pay attention to your thoughts: Did seeing or thinking about a certain food have an effect? What were you thinking about? Notice your conscious thoughts, as well as the ones you may have ignored. How are

you feeling? How did the feelings change as you came closer and closer to overeating? Were you experiencing a sense of deprivation, either physically or emotionally?

> Come up with one thing that you might do differently. If you find yourself becoming overwhelmed or discouraged, let go and return to your breath, refocusing as a detached, objective observer. As you continue to breathe fully and comfortably, return to watching the events, thoughts, and feelings that occurred as you came closer to overeating. Make a mental note of the possible triggers.

> Let go of that place and time, and let yourself refocus on your breath. Let go of any tension that cropped up, and simply ride with the flow of your breath, secure in the knowledge that you're putting together the pieces of the puzzle that will help you regain control over your eating. Now bring your attention back to the room, and when you're ready, open your eyes.

REFLECTION

> Did you find this exercise to be stressful? Why or why not?

> What triggers did you discover behind your overeating?

> What are some alternative ways to handle these triggers, rather than overeating? (Remember, there's a difference between eating and overeating! It's okay to use food for comfort sometimes.)

Week 6

DAY 1: MINDFULLY EATING FRUITS AND VEGETABLES

Just because a food is good for you doesn't mean you should stuff yourself with it to the point of discomfort. A plate of veggies is undoubtedly beneficial to your body, but you still need to learn to stop eating when you've reached a comfortable level of fullness. And you still need to figure out what you really want, even when you're eating healthy foods: "Am I in the mood for a banana or an apple? Celery or carrot sticks?" It's not necessarily problematic to eat both an apple and a banana, but there may be an overarching issue: If you eat both, it may be because you're not truly in touch with what your body is telling you it wants.

1. Prepare a plate of healthy snack foods, including fruit (such as orange and apple slices, berries, and chunks of pineapple and melon) and veggies of several colors and flavors (such as baby carrot sticks, cherry tomatoes, red or green pepper slices, and sugar snap peas). Make sure you use fresh produce.

2. Move into a mindful meditative state for a few moments, slowing down your breathing. Rate how physically hungry you are, then determine how you know this. Next, rate how full you are right now, being aware of how you know.

3. Take a few moments to look at the food. Choose three of the foods, including at least one fruit and one vegetable. Consider which looks most appealing, but also try to include one that you're not sure of. If the pieces are small, you can place more than one of each on your plate. Stop and consider how you made these choices.

4. Which flavor would you prefer at this moment? Reflect on how you made this choice. Pick up a piece of the fruit or vegetable, and notice its shape and color. Think about where this food came from and how it came to you. Bring the food to your lips, smell it, and feel its texture against your mouth.

5. Bite into the food, and chew it slowly. Rate the pleasure of the taste on a scale of 1 to 10, noticing how much you're enjoying the food. Continue to eat the rest of the first food in this way. Does the flavor change? Stop when you've finished eating all of the first food on your plate, or when you no longer want any more. Again, rate your hunger and fullness.

6. Reflect on which food you would like to eat next and then take a little bit of it, considering how you made this choice. Look at this food, notice its shape and color, and smell it. Feel the texture

against your lips—how is it different from the first food? Place it in your mouth, slowly chew it, and notice the burst of flavor in your mouth. Continue to eat the food mindfully, and note any differences in pleasure and satisfaction between this and the first food. Stop eating when you have finished this food or no longer enjoy it.

7. Take a moment to appreciate the food you've eaten, and rest your hand on your stomach. Be aware of your sense of fullness, as well as your hunger and satisfaction. Then bring your awareness back to your breath and back to the room, and gently open your eyes.

REFLECTION

> Did you want to continue eating? Did this exercise feel difficult? What was surprising? Interesting?

> How do you feel about not being asked to eat the third type of food on your plate? (If you'd like to, you can do so now—just do so mindfully!)

> How was this similar or different from the chips and cookies exercise?

> This exercise builds five skills: awareness of hunger, fullness, taste satiety, satisfaction, and making choices. Which were easier, and which were harder?

DAY 2: MINDFULLY EATING A MEAL

So far, you've mastered the mindful bite. Now you're ready to tackle the mindful *meal*—preferably with friends or family and with multiple types of foods to choose from. Hint: Pick a few friends who know about your weight-loss goals, ask everyone to bring a dish or two, and set up the food buffet-style. Before you dive in, plan to do the following to get maximum benefit from this exercise.

1. Start with a mini meditation (you don't have to close your eyes!) and rate your current level of hunger. Don't forget to pay attention to how you know this.

2. Survey all of the food on the table before taking anything. This is a core practice for cultivating balance, because there will often be more choices than you can eat.

3. Plan to go back for seconds. Think of Round 1 as a chance to sample your options, while Round 2 will consist of the foods you most enjoyed, and perhaps some new ones. You're not going for dessert just yet! If there is a selection of desserts, go at least twice to the dessert table, taking the same approach.

4. Leave food on your plate. Deciding *not* to clean your plate may sound like an exercise in deprivation, but this actually builds flexibility into your eating experience: You can decide which foods you like most and which you like least, and then you can practice using your inner experience as a guide for when to stop eating, rather than automatically scraping up every last bite.

5. Eat the first half of your meal in silence. Although eating mindfully doesn't have to mean zipping your lips—in fact, one of your goals is to learn to be mindful even in social situations—try to stay silent and focused on your eating experience during the first half of your meal, if possible. That way, you can notice the pleasure of eating, any thoughts or feelings that pop up, and how this differs from your normal experience of social eating, which often veers into mindless territory. Check in with yourself at least once during the conversation period: How's your hunger level? Is your taste satisfaction decreasing? How full is your stomach? Do you feel satisfied? Do you feel pleasure?

REFLECTION

> Did you successfully stop eating at the satiety level you wanted to? How did you do this?

> Were there any differences between which foods you thought you'd like and which you actually wanted more of?

> How did the social environment impact your ability to be aware of your eating?

> Was it hard for you to leave food on your plate? What thoughts came up about this?

DAY 3: MINDFULLY EATING AT A BUFFET

Now wait a few days, but take the skills you practiced to eating at a restaurant buffet. You may feel hesitant to even consider eating at a buffet: Not only are you confronted with an enormous number of options, but you're also battling the impulse to "get your money's worth," which often leads you to eat plate after plate of high-calorie foods. Another risk factor: You have little idea of what foods to expect, making it difficult to plan your choices ahead of time. This leaves you vulnerable to impulsive eating, especially if you're socializing while dining out.

Instead of avoiding it, view the challenging setting of a buffet as an opportunity to experiment with different food choices and to apply all of the skills you've learned. Don't forget to use the guidelines from the previous mindful-meal exercise (Week 6, Day 2, on page 256): Survey the available foods before dishing anything out, plan to "taste test" foods and then go back for seconds, and leave some food on your plate. This is a chance to be picky and eat only the dishes you really enjoy.

During the second half of your meal, you can chat with your partner or friends while trying to stay in a thoughtful state of mind.

Once you mindfully approach the buffet—even the inexpensive kind that's dominated by cheap carbs—you may be surprised to find some pretty reasonable options. You'll almost always have access to a salad bar, lean meats and seafood, and fresh fruit. Those are the cornerstones of any healthy-eating plan. But you can—and should—scan the other dishes; this can be a prime opportunity to sample more indulgent foods in small amounts, without anyone urging you to overdo it.

Once you grab a plate, you'll most likely realize that you've developed the skills you need to conquer the buffet, instead of letting it defeat you. As you survey the food for the first, second, or third time, observe your reactions.

> > Does your "craving" or "temptation" meter go up when you see certain foods? How does this change once you've sampled some of the foods?

> How can you use this setting to cultivate your inner gourmand?

> How hungry are you? How full?

REFLECTION

> Did you experience anxiety during the buffet dinner? Did this dissipate over the course of the meal?

> Did you use your inner experiences of hunger and satiety awareness to manage the buffet? Did this help you avoid overeating?

> What was the most difficult part of this experience? The most satisfying?

Postscript: After the Program

DAY 1: CHECK-IN

By now, you've probably made progress toward your goals, and often this progress comes in the form of small shifts in a positive direction. You're beginning to see that change does not occur all at once, but is instead an ongoing series of little steps taken one at a time. Hopefully, you've seen that it's not "all or nothing"—that you can have a bad day or two without it meaning that you've failed. Becoming mindful is a gradual, continual process that you'll stick with long after you've finished reading this book.

The tools you've learned are relatively simple: meditating daily in order to deepen your self-awareness, eating mindfully, and finding other ways to deal with difficult issues. As you continue practicing these skills, you'll gain more and more control over your eating. In fact, Dr. Kristeller's research has shown a direct relationship between people's frequency of mindfulness practice and their improvements in creating more balance and a sense of self-control surrounding eating. Each type of practice—regular meditation, eating-related meditation, and mini meditations—seemed to be related to greater success; all three together predicted the most change, including weight loss. And note that bringing mindfulness to eating doesn't mean that you have to eat slowly all of the time or to savor every bite. You might mindfully choose the best amount to eat for a meal and then quickly eat it before an important meeting, or you might just check in on your full-ness during a big meal so you don't really overdo it.

> As you continue implementing what you've learned, what do you anticipate being the greatest challenge? Is there a vacation or holiday coming up? A new job? Fears about slipping back into an old pattern? Jot down your concerns.

_____

_____

_____

_____

_____

> How can you make these situations seem more manageable?

_____

_____

_____

_____

_____

DAY 2: MAINTAINING AND CONTINUING CHANGE

Just as weight-loss ups and downs are inevitable, so are fluctuations in how mindful or balanced you are in your relationship with eating and food. Some days, tough emotions may drive you back to old habits, or you may simply start to fall back into some lifelong patterns of eating. But instead of seeing your slipups as failures, view them as opportunities to explore why a particular situation was a challenge. The goal here is not to be constantly policing your eating, but to become more relaxed yet balanced about it.

Generate a list of the obstacles you've noticed in maintaining the weight you've lost. Examples may include:

> **"I've changed my eating and am exercising, but I'm dissatisfied with the amount of my weight loss."**
>
> **"I'm slowly going back to old habits and worry that all of this work has been for nothing."**
>
> **"I thought I'd get more support from my boyfriend, but he keeps complaining that I'm not buying chips anymore."**
>
> **"I don't have time to prepare healthier meals."**
>
> **"I've noticed my motivation declining—I just want to eat mindlessly sometimes."**

Write down a few of your struggles here:

1. _____

_____

_____

2. _____

_____

_____

3. _____

_____

_____

4. _____

_____

_____

As trying as these challenges can be, you may find them easier to accept if you view creating a new relationship with food as a process of gradual change. Think about it this way: If you moved to a new town, it would certainly take more than a few weeks before you felt at home. As you continue working toward your goals, it's important to maintain a sense of exploration, openness, and willingness to try new things.

A big part of this process is accepting setbacks. Weight-loss obstacles create a gap between what we want or expect and the present outcome. It's perfectly natural to feel disappointed, frustrated, angry, hopeless, and even depressed when we encounter setbacks. What's critical is the way you respond: You can throw in the towel and give up, or you can continue to work with the difficult reality of changing your eating behavior. Sometimes, when you're tempted to quit, it's helpful to think about *why* you want to lose weight—for example, because you want to improve your family life, to boost your confidence, or to protect your health.

> Take a moment to reflect. Sit quietly and see if you can recall the intention you originally had when you decided to try this program. How did you feel in the beginning? Perhaps you were hopeful, serious, worried about your health, or tired of feeling embarrassed about your body. Whatever your reason, you wanted to direct your life away from what was distressing or harmful and toward something different.

> Center yourself, become aware of your breath, and see if you can sense this intention more fully. After a minute, try to sense the care you have toward yourself—to make changes to your eating, and perhaps to improve other parts of your life, as well. Appreciate the hard work you've already done. You hung in there. Sense the feeling of caring for yourself, whether that just means not being hard on yourself, letting up a little, or taking small steps to do what's best for you.

> Return to your breath. As you inhale, say to yourself, "As I work with new challenges," and as you exhale, say to yourself, "may I let go of expectations." Repeat this for several breaths.

> Notice your expectations: "I should have lost so much weight by now." "I shouldn't ever eat out of control." Use the sensation of letting go of the

breath to let go of your critical expectations. Expectations may be a simple goal, or you can use unmet expectations as ammunition against yourself. Let go of using expectations as a way to beat yourself up.

> Now bring your attention back to your breath, and sit in silence for 2 minutes. Then, as you breathe in, say to yourself, "As I sense my intention to care for myself," and as you breathe out, say to yourself, "may I let go of self-blame." Repeat these phrases several times. Notice self-blame; criticism; stubbornness of not wanting to let go. See if you can let go even for a moment, while paying attention to how tight your grip is.

> Return to your breathing for 2 minutes, then inhale and say to yourself, "As I sense my limits," and as you exhale, say to yourself, "may I let go of my impatience." Repeat for a few breaths. What does it feel like to respect your own rhythm? To let go of the extra pressure? To take the step that is doable at this moment? To let go of harshness and impatience?

> Bring your attention back to your breath, then gently open your eyes.

Boldface page references indicate photographs. <u>Underscored</u> references indicate boxed text.